The Oat Bran Miracle

Dr Pierre Dukan

The Oat Bran Miracle

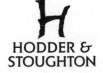

HODDER &
STOUGHTON

First published in Great Britain in 2013 by Hodder & Stoughton
An Hachette UK company

1

Copyright © Dr Pierre Dukan 2013

A CIP catalogue record for this title is available from the British Library

Trade Paperback ISBN 978 1 444 75695 1
Ebook ISBN 978 1 444 75793 4

Typeset in Celeste by Hewer Text UK, Ltd

Printed and bound by Clays Ltd, St Ives plc

Hodder & Stoughton policy is to use papers that are natural, renewable
and recyclable products and made from wood grown in sustainable
forests. The logging and manufacturing processes are expected to
conform to the environmental regulations of the country of origin.

Hodder & Stoughton Ltd
338 Euston Road
London NW1 3BH

www.hodder.co.uk

Contents

Contents

PART III: OAT BRAN RECIPES

Preface

How oat bran came into my life

Oat bran appeared in my life through one of the doors that goes straight to my heart – my daughter Maya.

Maya was then a teenager and, like all other teenagers nowadays, she thought she was a little too plump, so she would occasionally ask me, her nutritionist father, for help. Of course what she wanted was a miracle diet, a diet that would sort everything out in just a few days.

One morning I found her rummaging through the cupboards and the fridge searching for something satisfying to eat. She looked ready to make quite a feast of it, knowing full well she would have regrets afterwards. She did me the honour of asking me to choose something for her.

'What if I made you a pancake?' The word pancake struck just the right chord with my daughter – and who doesn't enjoy a pancake? Do you know many people who can tell you with complete equanimity, 'I do not like pancakes'? Round, golden, crispy yet melt-in-the mouth, sweet or savoury: our mouths start watering at the thought of pancakes as our minds conjure up enjoyable memories of pancake days and childhood teatimes. Pancakes belong in that category where food is a present and recipes a gift. Preparing them takes a little time and this in itself can be special and enjoyable. Try this out by asking a child or adult who is dear to you the question, 'What if I made you a pancake?' Immediately you will see their eyes light up and a big smile spread across their face.

While searching for some flour, I came across a packet of oat bran I had brought back from the United States, attracted by its claim that it was 'good for the heart'.

In no time at all, the frying pan was warming, three drops of oil had been added and wiped off with kitchen paper so that just enough remained to stop our pancake from sticking.

Carried away by the inspiration of the moment, I broke an egg, added some low-fat fromage frais and, acting on some secret and intuitive impulse, I grabbed the small packet of oat bran staring down at me from the shelf.

And I mixed it all together.

Leaning over my shoulder, my daughter opened the sweetener and sprinkled in a little of the white powder.

We whisked it together and at the last moment I added some milk to bind the mixture and a few drops of vanilla for taste.

And then we started cooking. The mixture went into the hot pan, two to three minutes for each side, and we ended up with a lovely, golden pancake. It was a good size and slightly thicker than a 'traditional' one.

We turned the pancake out on to our best white dining plate, one of the ones reserved for entertaining and which we also associate with eating blinis and pancakes. Maya lingered over every mouthful, took a second helping and could not get over being able to eat with such pleasure but without a guilty conscience. And I have to admit that I too enjoyed our delicious treat.

What happened afterwards? This recipe was to become part of the bedrock of my slimming method and one of the three pillars of its stabilization programme.

Now is perhaps the right time to recap on how, over the years, I developed and improved the Dukan method.

I had the good fortune to be the person who devised the first protein-based diet in France. This was at a time when it was thought that getting people to lose weight was an end in itself and that, once a person got down to the right weight, all that was needed to keep it off was a minimum amount of willpower.

I was young at the time and I went along with this naïve belief, proud of having devised a diet that got away from the traditional calorie-counting in low-calorie diets because my patients could now eat the 72 high-protein foods I allowed them, without any portion control or calculation.

Very quickly, I was forced to think again and add alternating days that included vegetables.

This new 'Cruise' phase meant patients could quickly attain their target weight, without feeling tired and with minimum frustration.

When I noticed that my patients were soon regaining the weight they had lost, drawn back to ingrained bad habits and by the appeal of comfort foods, I had to change my tune for a second time.

So that all my patients' hard work did not go to waste, I then added a Consolidation phase, a barrier of no return to prevent any weight rebound. Drawing on my experience and observation of post-dieting and early weight regain, I worked out that this period needed to last five days for every pound lost.

The method was already much improved; weight regain became less common and occurred much later on. However, it was still happening too frequently for my liking.

I then took the decision that gave my diet a whole new dimension, turning it into a lasting, complete programme. I introduced a permanent Stabilization phase based on three simple, strong, effective, not-too-frustrating but non-negotiable measures, including the famous protein Thursdays.

The slimming part of my diet – that is, the first two phases, Attack then Cruise – is built around two main components: lean animal proteins (meat and fish) and plant proteins that are low in sugars and high in fibre, as well as green vegetables.

This diet works and has legitimacy because it is what the first humans, our hunter-gatherer ancestors, started eating. Although we are 21st-century city dwellers, whose way of life and culture is shaped by our digital age, our bodies and our physiology have remained very close to that of the first humans. Since the conditions that give rise to the birth of a species are always in symbiosis with its environment, I have constructed my diet so that this throwback to our origins removes as much frustration as possible from the task the slimmer faces.

Today it has become a comprehensive method and, as immodest as it may appear, to the best of my knowledge this diet is the simplest, most natural and most effective slimming regime there is and the one that offers you irreversible weight loss. In a nutshell, it is the diet I would have prescribed to my daughter if she had really needed to lose weight.

For over 30 years I drew on my experience of working daily with weight problems, continually developing and honing this diet. However, for a long time it had one weakness – very few carbohydrates and no cereals or starchy foods at all during the Attack and Cruise phases.

When starting the diet most of my patients felt no need for carbohydrates as the amount of weight they were initially shedding made them euphoric. However, as they persisted with the diet, the final few pounds would take the longest to shift and they would end up hankering after crusty bread, nourishing pasta, potatoes or rice. In short, one or other of those foods that both satisfy hunger and provide comfort. We no doubt crave these foods because they take us back to our early childhood tastes and habits (children are huge fans of chips, mash, pasta and hunks of bread). These high-carbohydrate foods are like 'magnets drawing you back to past pleasures'. More than their nutritional value, it is their emotional power that makes them so attractive and so swift to guarantee us pleasure and satiety. I will return to this crucial psychological factor later on.

Having found its way into my authorized foods sanctuary, oat bran lifted this restriction on carbohydrates and my diet worked considerably better and over a longer period of time.

The patients I saw in my consultations were the first to benefit from it. Then the forums got hold of the discovery and oat bran turned into a slimming food. Today you only have to type 'Dukan galette' into Google to see that it gets thousands of hits.

A miracle?

When penned by a doctor, this word sounds strange, especially when it appears in the actual title of their book.

Why so much praise and enthusiasm for oat bran?

Because 'miracle' is quite simply the *mot juste*. Oat bran is indeed a sort of wonder; all the more so because the way it works, its effects and all it can achieve contrast so starkly with its modest appearance and inexpensiveness.

Oat bran is a foodstuff that plays a role in the four most important areas of health. Its work is direct, straightforward and scientifically proven on cholesterol – high levels of which can lead to blocked arteries and heart disease – and cancer, the two established killers of our modern age. It also works on two other major risk factors: diabetes and weight problems. Being overweight or obese will impact on cholesterol levels, cancer and diabetes.

What other medication or foodstuff can make such claims? My task is to convince you of my argument and this is why, among other reasons, I have written this book.

But, you will point out, it was not me who invented oat bran. A cure-all of this kind would have long since aroused the interest of dieticians, doctors, cardiologists, cancer and diabetes specialists. This is true, of course. However, they all viewed it only from their own narrow perspective, focusing solely on how it works within their particular specialist area.

American cardiologists see oat bran's importance as beyond dispute and companies that manufacture whole oat products, bran included, are allowed the wording 'good for the heart' on their packaging. The American Food and Drug Administration, well known for its strict criteria, has for the first time awarded this foodstuff 'nutraceutical' status.

Diabetes specialists acknowledge the role that soluble fibre – in oat bran and pectin – plays in slowing down the rate at which sugars are absorbed. Once it becomes stuck in soluble fibre, a simple sugar turns into a complex sugar so that as it enters the bloodstream our blood sugar level goes up less and at a slower rate.

Cancer specialists were the first to discover that all fibre, soluble and insoluble, helps protect the body from cancer, and all the more so as our diet becomes increasingly reliant on processed foods and products that our intestines are in no hurry to clear out.

Gastroenterologists know from experience that fibre, in particular soluble fibre, cannot be absorbed by the body. As this fibre soaks up water, it gives our stools bulk and volume which naturally keeps our bowel movements regular.

When listed together all these benefits do make oat bran seem like a panacea, but nobody got excited about them because each medical discipline used the bran in its own way for its own ends, thus keeping hidden just how useful it is.

For its full value to be recognized, this already impressive list of health benefits was not enough; it needed a 'weighty' argument, a key theme, one of burning interest. And I was able to provide this argument by revealing another way in which oat bran works physiologically, in another field of treatment – namely, weight and obesity problems. This may appear a less dramatic field of treatment but these problems are spreading across the world while medicine looks on helplessly and does little to stop the epidemic.

In fact, as far as many doctors are concerned, putting on weight within reasonable limits is not an illness. If anything it is taken as a sign of good health, the implication being that a body that takes full advantage of what it eats is far healthier than one which loses weight for no reason. They only start to take an interest in weight problems once these have become sufficiently developed and long-standing to give rise to pathological complications.

However, when the average person worries about being overweight, health considerations are rarely uppermost in their mind. For them, putting on weight means a shameful appearance, a physical burden, an ordeal that is hard to bear, and for the vast majority of overweight people this results in intense suffering.

Anything that may ease this suffering is of huge import, so I am appealing to everyone involved with weight issues – doctors, journalists, chefs, caterers, food manufacturers, health professionals and, first and foremost, anyone who is overweight – to fully grasp the miraculous scope of all that oat bran can do.

This bran which is so exceptional is no simple foodstuff – it is a complete food concept.

It would be useful therefore to turn our attention to oat bran's active substance, its soluble fibre, because it is this fibre that explains and underpins all the many ways in which oat bran helps to prevent disease.

This will not be some complicated, impenetrable and tedious chemistry lesson. I will stick to simple, clear facts; the results speak for themselves anyway.

I will then, of course, look at how oat bran works on weight, its fascinating role in reducing calories as an antifood that actually induces 'calorie leakage'. This role would have had oat bran banished from our diets for ever in a world where there was not enough to eat, which lasted until the end of the 19th century. Nowadays, thanks to our food abundance and the paradoxically dire repercussions this has had on our health and happiness, oat bran is now something of a heaven-sent food – a slimming food but also a healthy food since it is particularly beneficial for anyone who dreads the threat of high cholesterol, has well-established diabetes or is developing diabetes or for whom it runs in the family.

Anyone with a family history of cancer, particularly cancer of the colon, and all those people whose bowels have become sluggish for lack of fibre and exercise will also find something of interest here.

Introduction

What is oat bran?

Oat bran fibre, where it all happens

In France, where bread is a sacred food, oats were considered a poor, inferior cereal, useless for bread-making and good only for feeding horses or filling mattresses.

In oats, as in wheat and most other cereals, there is the noble grain, a concentrated source of energy, and the husk that protects it, a little like the shell around an egg.

As far as nutrition is concerned, the energy provided by oats is concentrated in the grain where it is stored. Oat flour is made from oat grain – the traditional oat flakes or rolled oats. It is very important not to confuse bran with oatmeal or oat flakes.

As a rule we are mainly interested in the grain and its calories. However, what excites me is the 'non-foodstuff' part of the oats, the bran, the hardy, outer casing. Why is it a 'non-foodstuff'? Unlike ruminants and herbivores, we humans do not have the right enzymes to break down and absorb its long food chains.

What makes oat bran so special, and why it merits a whole book, is precisely because it passes right through our digestive tract, from the mouth where it soaks up saliva, via the stomach where it plays its role in filling us up to perfection to the colon. And throughout this journey it withstands every sort of physical and chemical treatment it encounters.

This soluble oat bran fibre, saturated with water and extremely viscous on contact, starts to perform its incredible role once it reaches the small intestine where our body extracts nutrients and calories from the food we eat. It is here that the famous oat bran miracle takes place.

What is in this casing, the bran that is so unusual and so precious? It is fibre but not just any old fibre.

In the vegetable kingdom, there are two sorts of fibre. Soluble fibre, which can dissolve in water and soak it up, and insoluble fibre. Brans from wheat and most other plants are insoluble. Oat bran is soluble in water as is the pectin in apples. Pectin fibre has similar properties but extracting it is far more difficult and costly and separating it from the fruit's sugars is even trickier.

Nevertheless, pectin guarantees the apple's medicinal potential, so aptly summed up in the English saying 'an apple a day keeps the doctor away'. This proves that the British have long known about the benefits of eating apples, which have since been confirmed by modern pharmacology.

Other insoluble fibre such as wheat bran is far less useful. It allays hunger, of course, and speeds up digestion, but it irritates sensitive colons and this limits its use.

Let us take a further look at oat bran's soluble fibre. How does it protect the body and why is it good for us?

Oat bran fibre is different because, being soluble, it is able to soak up liquids, and on contact with them can turn into a gel with high viscosity. This precious fibre acts like a sponge. Its sponge-like structure, with its alveoli, can absorb up to 30 times its volume in water.

If you put some oat bran in water or milk you get a

mixture very similar to porridge, quite different from what you have if you use wheat bran, which settles at the bottom of the container. If you examine a drop of oat bran solution through a microscope you will see a lattice network of alveoli trapping the water inside the enclosed spaces. This is what happens, whatever liquid you dissolve the bran in.

In the digestive tract, the stomach opens into the small intestine which is a long, narrow canal ten or more metres – well over 30 feet – long, where the body obtains its nutrients and calories and every other substance that keeps it alive. Here is the interface between food and blood, the external world and the internal world.

The food has already been broken down by some initial chewing and the action of our salivary enzymes, before it is mechanically churned in the stomach's acidic environment. In the small intestine the chemicals in the bile then work on the food, cleaning out the fats while the pancreatic juice breaks down the long protein chains. This process is vital as food can only pass into the bloodstream if it has already been broken down into indivisible unit cells.

So proteins end up as amino acids, fats (lipids) as fatty acids and sugars (carbohydrates) in a pre-glucose state.

At this point, no recognizable trace of the food remains as the food bolus is now a sort of liquid pulp. This is the final stage and how thick or thin it is will depend on the food ingested and the quantity of liquid consumed. Now comes the crucial moment when at last the body can suck up these basic elements and use them to extract the energy and materials it needs to build and repair itself.

What happens if you add oat bran to this food bolus?

The constellation of alveoli opens out and the bran absorbs 30 times its initial volume. In these alveoli there will be nutrients and calories that have managed to find their way in but which get stuck and find it very hard to get out. They remain trapped in there.

This fibre and its load then pass through the small intestine. The small intestine will attempt to extract any nutritive juices but to little avail. Once the bran leaves the small intestine and moves into the large colon, the opportunity has been lost. The colon can no longer provide any calories; its role is restricted to slowly extracting water from the food bolus so that it becomes more solid and can turn into stools.

So when these stools are expelled from the colon and the body, they take with them most of the oat bran fibre along with its alveoli, now laden with nutrients and calories. A sponge that traps food and can prevent it from passing into the bloodstream – this is the marvellous way in which oat bran works.

We are now going to discover how this trapping ability works at the very root of all metabolic processes, for sugars as well as fats and proteins – namely, on all the calories they carry.

Part I:

A slimming food

Oat bran: your weight-loss friend

Oat bran is the only natural food that can claim to be a slimming food. If I go by my extensive personal experience and the thousands of people who have written about it on the internet, it is now possible to treat oat bran as not only a food that aids slimming but, perhaps even more so, as a food that helps us stabilize the weight we slim down to.

Although calorie loss through eating oat bran is only modest, it is nonetheless real and can be repeated without any danger.

Oat bran works in three ways:

- by removing a modest amount of the calories in your food, thereby reducing the total number assimilated;
- by soaking up water and increasing to 30 times its volume in your stomach, this mechanical action makes you feel full and satiated;
- by lending itself easily to an endless number of sweet and savoury dishes because of its consistency and flavour.

How oat bran sneaks away food and calories

Eating oat bran enables you to reduce the calories you extract from the food you consume. From this point of view, oat bran can be considered to be an anti-food. Its fibre comes out of your body containing more calories than when it went in. The oat bran sneaks these calories away from the food it comes into contact with, preventing them from passing into the bloodstream.

This process has so much going for it that we need to take a closer look.

In our mouths and stomachs, oat bran undergoes attack as it is assailed by acids. However, this does not alter its structure because our bodies do not have the right enzymes to digest it.

The food bolus around the bran becomes more fluid and once the pylorus (the orifice that connects the stomach with the entrance to the small intestine) opens up, the bran that has dissolved into the bolus moves with it into this sanctuary where exchanges take place between the body and the external world. Here the bran undergoes a twofold attack from the bile secreted by the liver and the pancreatic juice. After this chemical onslaught, the food bolus now only contains a mixture of the three universal nutrients – proteins, lipids and carbohydrates – completely broken down into their basic parts and ready to pass into the bloodstream. It is here that the oat bran fibre will play its part in intercepting their absorption; to put it simply, it blocks their way.

What happens to the proteins?

This nutrient which comes mostly from animals (meat, fish and by-products) but from plants, too, is made up of long chains with covalent bonds. Of all the bonds between elementary links, it is these bonds that put up the greatest resistance to being broken down.

A slimming food

Now is an opportune moment to explain to you one of the ways in which protein is so useful in a strategy to tackle weight problems. In the weight-loss method that I spent years developing, proteins are hugely important. The process of breaking down food chains into elementary links can vary widely between different foods and what it is that binds them together. This process can burn up 30 per cent of the calories the food contains. For example, a beefsteak containing 250 calories would take you almost 70 calories just to break down its long protein chains so that the amino acids could pass into your bloodstream. This means that your steak has become naturally leaner since now it will provide you with only 180 calories.

Using up calories in this way is what chemists call SDA, the 'Specific Dynamic Action', of food. For some sugars, which we call simple or fast-release sugars, this action is very low – a sugar cube easily dissolves and puts up little resistance to being digested. By the time it reaches the small intestine only two calories will have been used to break it down. Its dynamic action is 5 per cent and of the 40 calories contained in the cube, 38 will pass into the bloodstream as glucose. Complex or slow-release sugars, such as those in pasta, legumes, lentils and peas, put up more resistance; they pass into the bloodstream more slowly and to a lesser extent, so their action may be as high as 12 per cent. As for fat, its dynamic action is 10 per cent.

You can now understand why eating proteins is so important if you want to lose weight.

What is more, you should also realize that when you eat a piece of meat, fish or poultry the proteins that make up these foods all have a structure and a series of amino acids that is peculiar to each species. However, regardless of the species, its proteins are assembled from the same amino acids. There are 20 amino acids, of which eight are essential. The only thing that varies from one species to another is how they are arranged.

Once broken down and absorbed into the bloodstream, proteins that once came, for example, from a duck will be put back together in the order that is peculiar to human beings so that they become human proteins. If one day you were to be eaten by a lion, this lion would do the very same thing and would turn your human proteins into lion proteins. You should be aware, too, that this recomposition process of 'manufacturing' new proteins also uses up calories.

So keep in mind that the nutrient that works best in a slimming strategy is proteins and it is for this very reason that I made them the spearhead of my diet.

What happens to the sugars?

There are two sorts of sugars: simple (fast-release) sugars and complex (slow-release) sugars. Simple sugars are the ones that have a sweet, sugary taste. They are made up of a few basic molecules. Sucrose in table sugar, fructose in fruit and lactose in milk are the main sources.

Complex sugars are compounds with a great number

of molecules. These are the sugars found in cereals and starchy foods. They have long chains; this explains why it takes so long to break them down and why they are called slow-release sugars.

The final basic element is glucose. It is no surprise to see a person's blood sugar level go up or down depending on which sugary food is being eaten. Honey, breakfast cereals and white bread rush straight into the bloodstream, sending blood sugar levels soaring, whereas slow sugars pass into the bloodstream as they are being broken down, which means the blood sugar level increases only gradually and hyperglaecemic spikes are avoided.

These spikes are dangerous for our bodies, and especially so for diabetics and people who are overweight. This is because when glucose concentration in the blood exceeds one gram per litre, it becomes irritating, then aggressive and finally toxic for all our arteries. This is equally true for the arterioles as for the main arteries and it has the same impact as putting sugar in your car's petrol tank. To protect itself from this danger, the body gets the pancreas to produce insulin. Insulin is a natural hormone whose job is to get rid of excessive blood glucose by driving it into two places where it is naturally stored – our liver and our muscles.

A diabetic person has a deficient pancreas that does not secrete enough insulin and it struggles increasingly to sponge up this excess glucose. Whenever there is too much sugar in the blood, this sugar will slowly but surely damage whatever is containing it: the heart and the vessels of all the organs that are supplied with blood, the kidneys, eyes, lower limbs, brain and so on. This is why diabetes can be so hugely damaging. Unfortunately it takes hold gradually and insidiously and, just like a time bomb, once it explodes, it explodes everywhere at the same time.

There are two reasons why insulin makes us put on weight.

- Sending glucose to the liver where it is stored as glycogen results in insulin making it easier for the body to store fat. The more insulin there is in our blood, the more fat we accumulate and store.
- Insulin makes us feel hungry; snacking on anything sugary suddenly raises our blood sugar level and forces the pancreas to protect our body with very high quantities of insulin and this keeps us feeling hungry. It really is a vicious circle.

However, oat bran fibre is able to slow down the rate at which sugars pass into the bloodstream and by doing this it slows down insulin production. It protects the diabetic's pancreas and helps carbohydrate fans limit their weight gain.

When digestion is over, some glucose lingers on in the bolus in your intestines, getting ready to pass through into your blood. It is here in this sugary juice that the bran gets to work spinning its delaying web. The glucose passes through far more slowly and those glycaemic spikes that wear out the pancreas are avoided.

What happens to the fats?

The third nutrient dealt with during digestion is fats – nature being thrifty, there are only three nutrients! We eat lipids or fats in the form of animal or vegetable fats, either pure as in oils or hidden away in foods such as cakes, biscuits, delicatessen products and cheeses. The digestion process concentrates on reducing fats down to fatty acids, the basic compounds.

Incidentally, you should bear in mind that whether it be animal or vegetable, fat is a nutrient that enables us to store the most calories in the least volume. Fat from plants or animals is a calorie supply that has been saved and stored away just like your own fat. So whenever you eat lipids, remember you are eating fat belonging to others, whether they are animals or plants – the very same sort of fat that you are trying to lose by dieting. So it is obvious that if you want to lose fat the first thing you must do is to significantly reduce your consumption of fat from other species.

Let's come back to the fatty acids, produced as the fats are finally broken down. Once they arrive in the small intestine, ready to pass through the mucous membrane and into the bloodstream, the oat bran fibre traps them in the mesh of its viscous gel, limiting what can be absorbed as the bran manages to take some of the fatty acids away with it into the stools.

In the end, the oat bran fibre has been there all along with the food while it was being transformed physically and chemically. Once it reaches the small intestine, on contact with the amino acids, fatty acids and glucose, the fibre forms a solution with the food in the bolus.

Throughout the digestive process, the oat bran fibre has time to open out, relax and form really large vacuoles that soak up water and these three nutrients. Once you realize that one tablespoonful of oat bran absorbs 30 times its volume, you can start to imagine these thousands upon thousands of vacuoles saturated with calories and nutrients.

As the stomach ends, the small intestine starts and extends for over ten metres. When there is no oat bran, most of what has been broken down and reduced to a state of basic elements passes through into the bloodstream. There is no filter or sieve here, only a system that sucks up the food; how hard it sucks depends on how hungry you are and how much energy you require. The food passes through the small intestine as if it were travelling along a conveyor belt. The body only has so much time to help itself, so it eagerly hoovers up everything it can extract.

It is here that oat bran works its miracle

The oat bran's viscous vacuoles hold on to the nutrients and calories it has soaked up and so they withstand the body's powerful sucking. Since the bran cannot be assimilated, it cannot be sucked up and so it is able to keep on travelling until it reaches the end of the small intestine.

The fibre, along with the calories it is carrying with it, then moves into the colon. This is now the large intestine and its only function is to drain off liquid from any waste and residue left after the food bolus has passed through the small intestine. The colon pumps away the water; the remains of the food bolus get dried out and transformed into solid stools.

Here another property of this incredible fibre comes to the fore. Just as the oat bran fibre withstood being sucked up by the small intestine, it similarly resists being absorbed into the colon and it hangs on to some of the water it is carrying. By doing this, it ensures that there is some moisture in the stools, which means that they are of a certain volume and it is easier for them to move through the colon, thus avoiding constipation.

Lastly, as it reaches the end of the large colon, having withstood the destruction and absorption process in both intestines, the oat bran fibre residue and its contents are expelled from the body in the stools.

Water is found in these stools, slightly more than when there is no oat bran, and most importantly there are nutrients and the 'stolen' calories. When stools containing soluble fibre from pectin or oat bran are analyzed, it is beyond doubt that they contain more calories than when there is no pectin or oat bran. We are therefore entitled to affirm that these calories have been removed from the food ingested after it was digested and that this in no way detracted from the pleasure taken in eating the food, nor was digestion in any way disrupted. A minor calorie hijacking has taken place. It is indeed minor, but it can be repeated at every mealtime throughout a weight-loss diet and in particular during that crucial period when you are stabilizing your weight, and you can do this for as long as you are striving to stay at the weight you have successfully slimmed down to.

Some people will say, 'If the bran can take with it calories and nutrients, it must also be taking with it mineral salts and vitamins in the same manner – and perhaps even medication.'

Yes, this is correct. However, as I have just stated, only small quantities are expelled and these are not enough to alter the balance of vitamins and medication within the food bolus. Nevertheless, it is useful to be aware of this if you are very sensitive, so that your food intake can be adjusted accordingly.

For example, anyone who suffers a lot from spasmophilia and tetanic spasms, and is hyper-sensitive to the magnesium content in food, simply needs to make sure that their magnesium intake is increased. This can easily be done by drinking two glasses of water with a high magnesium content every day.

Post-menopausal women with osteoporosis are advised to increase dairy product consumption slightly and drink water with a high calcium content.

With regard to vitamins and potassium, any losses are so tiny that unless you know you have a slight deficiency there is usually nothing gained by taking vitamin and mineral supplements.

Finally, for anyone following a low-fat weight-loss diet over an extended period it may be useful to monitor vitamin E levels. To offset eating a considerable amount of oat bran, all it takes is one teaspoon of sunflower oil per week. Vitamin A intake is taken care of by the carotene in vegetables; vitamin D is provided by oily fish and the sun.

When it comes to medication, absorption drops so very slightly that it has no impact on the doses generally taken. However, since there are fanatical oat bran devotees who are capable of eating excessive amounts – I have known patients who would eat a packet a day – if the medication is compulsory and important it is advisable to take it one hour after eating any oat bran.

These minor drawbacks are easily circumvented and only apply to a very few people who eat excessive quantities of oat bran and are on special medication (who should speak to their GP), so they should not distract us from how enormously useful this foodstuff is. Oat bran is the most effective among our wealth of human foods, and also more effective than a great number of food supplements and even some medicine.

So oat bran's soluble fibre carries out this rare operation of sneaking away calories, deducting a tax from the energy we consume. We can have our food intake whittled away and our energy intake modestly but quite definitely trimmed down, and it is oat bran fibre that makes this wonder possible.

As I conclude this chapter on how oat bran makes a major contribution to weight management, I would like to point out that today within the online Dukan community there is an impressive number of websites, blogs and forums where helpful people generously describe in great detail what they know about oat bran and what they have been able to do with it. Many write a simple description, others provide photos and some even post video clips. If you need any help, take a look at our website, which has the official forum and all the recipes. And should you need daily monitoring, you only have to enter the code HOD30 and a warm welcome will be extended to you along with our special terms.

Oat bran in the Dukan Diet

I have already described to you the main phases in the Dukan Diet, the food part of the method that its followers have decided to name after me. This is how I advise you to use oat bran throughout the diet so that you get the very best results:

- During the Attack phase, short but lightning quick, producing highly motivating results, I advise one tablespoonful of oat bran daily.
- During the Cruise phase, which comes afterwards and takes you straight to your True Weight, I recommend a daily dose of one to two tablespoonfuls, depending on how much weight you aim to lose.

You can eat it how you want – stirred into milk or water, sprinkled over salads, into omelettes, as a sweet galette or savoury blinis, or you can make bread or pizza dough with it.

Since the oat bran galette became a part of my diet, it has enjoyed continued success, with a great many women trying it and coming up with their own different ways of making it. Their creativity, and their support for others with weight problems, has inspired them to send me their recipes. I have included most of these at the end of the book, and if you come up with a new one then please send it to me too so that I can add it to the collection.

The Consolidation phase and then the long-term Stabilization phase are trickier.

I consider that weight has been successfully lost if, and only if, it is kept off for five years. The weight you slim down to is achieved after a great struggle and generally it remains unstable and at risk if the reasons that caused the excess weight are not sorted out. Your Stabilization weight will always remain an artificial weight and it will carry on fluctuating, more so than a normal weight would.

If these fluctuations are slight they should not cause you any concern. It is just your body breathing normally and such 'breathing' will vary according to your life's seasons and cycles.

However, once weight starts going back on and exceeds half of what was originally lost, then this is clearly a relapse. Once all the weight originally lost has been regained, this is now a 'repeat offence' and if weight regain exceeds the weight you were at when slimming started this is a repeat offence with the beginnings of a step-by-step descent into obesity. To prevent or counter this phenomenon, so common that some experts consider it totally inevitable, I have built this Stabilization phase around a trio of measures that are simple, concrete, precise and effective but indivisible and non-negotiable. When combined, these three measures can on their own offer long-term protection to this vulnerable stabilization weight. The longer the stabilization period lasts, based on these new habits, the more permanently established this protection becomes against relapses and repeat offending.

A slimming food

Controlling your True Weight over a very long period – if possible over a lifetime – hinges on three measures:

- Protein Thursdays – a sentinel day that stands guard over you, a day when you eat only high-protein foods such as meat, fish, poultry, eggs and low-fat dairy products, and drink lots of water.
- You contract to give up once and for all using lifts or escalators and to walk for 20 minutes a day.
- Three tablespoonfuls of oat bran every day for as long as you want to stabilize, and possibly for life in those tricky cases where a tendency to repeat offend has already become apparent.

How oat bran works on appetite and satiety

If oat bran's effect on appetite produces less amazing results than the way it soaks up food and calories, it is nevertheless pronounced and very useful. All known plant fibre has the ability to soak up water and of all fibre oat bran fibre works best. It does a wonderful job of making us feel full.

For anyone who wants to lose weight or keep their weight under control, this mechanical process comes into its own when it takes place inside the stomach.

Feeling hunger and the degree to which the stomach is full are directly related. An empty stomach complains when it is famished; when it is full we feel satiated and once it is too full we start to feel sick. Between the two ends of the spectrum lies a whole range of sensations and behaviour patterns correlating to just how full we are.

How does this mechanical process of satiety work?

When we fill our stomachs, the stomach walls are stretched and the little nerve rami that run through the stomach are distended. The brain receives a message that these sensory receptors are being distended; it assimilates this information and reacts to it by producing a sensation of satiety.

As surprising as it may seem, this is very similar to what gastric band surgery sets out to achieve.

The idea of inserting a gastric band in an obese person's stomach is to partially seal it off. The gastric band creates an obstacle that prevents the stomach from filling up. It then takes just a few mouthfuls to fill up what remains of the stomach, so that reaching satiety or even the point of feeling sick happens incredibly quickly. Gastric bands work with quantities and not with what type of food is being eaten.

What can be the connection between how a gastric band works and how oat bran works?

Given how soluble oat bran fibre is and its ability to absorb and become saturated, it only takes a few table-spoonfuls of oat bran to fill up a considerable part of the stomach. Follow my calculations carefully: each table-spoonful of oat bran weighs a little over 12g. Given that the bran absorbs 30 times its volume in liquid, this trans-forms the weight of a single tablespoonful into 450g. Three tablespoonfuls a day make 1350g which is capable of filling up a substantial part of the stomach. Which, if you think about it, fits with what gastric band surgery is trying to do. However, oat bran is less intrusive and, most importantly, it offers you the pleasure of a sweet, substantial cereal that can be used and enjoyed in a thou-sand recipes.

When eaten with a meal, each tablespoonful of oat bran turns into a nice supple pellet that spends a long time in the stomach, taking its time to get thoroughly mixed up and combined with the food, until it is expelled when the stomach opens up. All big eaters, with impatient appetites that are difficult to satisfy, are well advised to eat some oat bran at the start of a meal. However, this is only recom-mended if they drink water at the same time, otherwise there will not be enough liquid for the bran to soak up, so the feeling of satiety will not be achieved.

Oat bran can also make a useful snack if you feel the need to nibble at something in between meals. A sweet or savoury galette is a most delicious and perfectly appropriate way of eating it if you want to 'graze'.

Oat bran: a pleasure food

The icing on the cake is that as well as sneaking away calories and inducing satiety, oat bran fibre also turns out to have a highly enjoyable flavour and consistency. This fortunate feature means that we need have no qualms about introducing our exceptional cereal into diets that are low in starchy foods and cereals to offset any frustration at not being able to eat this sort of carbohydrate.

The bran's solubility and capacity to absorb liquid makes it pleasantly chewy and nice and creamy. Many people have got into the habit of making oat bran porridge with cinnamon, vanilla, coffee or orange blossom flavoured milk. Others prefer it plain, enjoying its delicate yet homely cereal flavour. There are others, and I include myself among them, who love eating oat bran in pancakes and galettes that are crispy yet melt in the mouth.

The basic recipe for my famous oat bran galettes could not be simpler. You take a whole egg (or just the egg white if you prefer), one heaped tablespoon of oat bran and one tablespoon of fromage frais. Milk, quark and skimmed milk powder may be used instead of fromage frais, depending on how light you want your mixture and how thick you like your galette. Ideally, if you have time, you would separate the egg, whisk up the white until stiff and then add the yolk. This makes the galette even lighter and smoother. Using a whole egg makes the galette more filling.

Let us briefly turn our attention again to the idea of frustration; it is part and parcel of any hard work and therefore of any diet. If you are finding the lack of carbohydrates really tough and you have cravings and urges, then go ahead and make up for not indulging them by increasing the number of galettes you have in a day. Some of my patients double up the doses and make themselves enormous galettes. They add a little salt and then they feast on delicious blinis with a double slice of smoked salmon, or sliced ham, turkey or chicken. Others sprinkle in some herbes de Provence or, the height of sophistication, some sesame seeds. What a treat!

At the end of this book you will find all sorts of recipes but why not try thinking up your own? Use oat bran to fit in with your own tastes and inclinations.

Before I discovered oat bran, my method relied on eating only high-protein foods and vegetables, alternating between them (so a day of pure proteins followed by a day of proteins combined with vegetables). Many of my patients desperately missed eating bread and starchy foods. Ever since oat bran took up its place in my method, I have noticed that sticking to my diet has become much easier. The results are just as impressive and stabilization is far longer-lasting. There is nothing surprising about this. By including oat bran in my diet, I introduced a first-rate pleasure and anti-frustration food.

I have always considered the Stabilization phase to be fundamental. Indeed, there would be no point at all in you forcing yourself to lose weight if once you reached your True Weight nothing was done to ensure that the pounds you have shed stayed off for good. Yet this is the Achilles heel in all diets. For over 60 years, for as long as we have been tackling weight problems, I have never come across a slimming method that establishes a Stabilization phase worthy of the name and that I could pay tribute to. By this I mean one with measures that are properly defined and easy to understand and apply, concrete but not too frustrating measures you would be happy to follow over the very long term. The majority of methods, even the most serious ones, finish up with some common-sense advice and simply appeal to you to exercise your willpower if you want to keep the weight off.

In my method, one of the cornerstones of the Stabilization phase is oat bran, as is 'contracting to give up taking lifts and escalators and walking for 20 minutes a day' (agreed to and carried out) and 'protein Thursdays' (a sentinel day to protect you, during which only Attack phase foods are eaten).

These three elements combined – protein Thursdays + stairs only and walking + oat bran – form the core of my Stabilization phase. This means anyone who embarks on my diet knows they stand a very serious chance of never, ever putting back on the weight they will manage to lose with the method.

After you have slimmed down, maintaining your weight is so terribly important, as much for the individual concerned as for weight problems statistics, that sticking to these three measures becomes easy to accept once people have had properly explained to them exactly what is at stake.

The easiest and most pleasant of these three rules is obviously taking three tablespoonfuls of oat bran daily.

I am on very good terms with former patients, who used to be overweight and who have now stabilized their weight once and for all. For the most part, they succeeded in doing this because they changed their lives and their new life made them sufficiently happy not to need to look to food for compensation. This simple happiness, often family-based, had altered their relationship with food. Now they eat when they need to feed themselves, allowing themselves occasionally a little 'treat for the taste buds' but always in moderation. Of those patients whose weight I deem to be permanently stabilized, a great many have stuck with the habit of eating oat bran, which for them has become a pleasure. When stabilization is built around adopting habits for good, oat bran is a great secret and a wonderful resource. It combines and enhances two pleasures, the pleasure of losing weight with that of enjoying eating.

This being the case, given my method and its restrictions, oat bran is the only carbohydrate food that may be included without hesitation as part of a weight-loss diet. Better still, it is the only carbohydrate food that ensures its success!

If you are one of those people who have unfortunately tried a succession of diets, you may well think there is something wrong with your hormones or metabolism.

Your problem is definitely more than just one of controlling your pleasure. If you can no longer bear the dreadful yo-yo effect, if you genuinely want to put all that behind you, then whatever you do, do not give up the pleasure of eating. Without pleasure, any diet is as good as doomed to failure. If you are a veteran of the weight battle remember this piece of advice: even with a restrictive diet include an element of pleasure, a life-line that will stop your project from foundering. To my mind, I have not found anything better than oat bran.

On many occasions during my career as a medical practitioner, I have looked after patients who for professional reasons have been in a tremendous hurry to lose weight – boxers before a match, who had to get back inside their weight category, jockeys who had to keep under a weight limit, movie stars, and dancers at the Opera House or with the Crazy Horse cabaret show.

Each time I find myself under pressure with this sort of emergency, I turn to oat bran. For one, two and even three days in the most urgent cases, I prescribe a double galette, using egg white only, four times a day; one in the morning, one for lunch, one in the afternoon and one for dinner. This is the quickest way I know of reaching a set target without frustration, fatigue or eroding muscle mass. It is of course imperative that these 'treatments' last only a very short time, that they are always occasional and driven by the circumstances.

I am a medical doctor and nutritionist and have had contact for a long time now with people who suffer terribly because they cannot live with their weight. This suffering is subjective and at times unrelated to how many pounds actually need to be lost, but for the most part it is intense, acute and awfully difficult to live with.

I very often see couples for consultations and meet obese husbands willing to help their wives follow a diet without it even crossing their mind that they should tackle their own obesity. Each person experiences what it is to be overweight in their own particular way.

During the past 30 years, within one generation, I have watched the world change and our Western lifestyle notch up its achievements as well as its afflictions. I am convinced, from working with my patients, that nowadays it is infinitely easier to put on weight and more difficult to take it off than it was three decades ago.

Why is this so?

The people that I help to lose weight lead lives that have changed so much, the women more so than the men. This new lifestyle is of course denser and richer, offering all sorts of things to stimulate and satisfy, but it is also more stressful and leaves us more vulnerable. Many men and women suffer from being obsessed with having to do and succeed at everything within a set timescale.

At the same time, a great number of man-made needs have found their insidious way into this new lifestyle, competing with our genuine needs and making these seem dull and ordinary so as to supplant them all the more easily.

You will want to know what is a genuine need and what is a false one.

A genuine need is a programmed need that we are driven to satisfy. It is both a desire that motivates us and a reward we experience as an enjoyable sensation we call pleasure.

For example, you are tempted by a lovely, beautifully cooked piece of sirloin steak or fish. You eat it and this gives you pleasure, a feeling of satisfaction and satiety. At the same time you are providing your body with the proteins you need to live, the amino acids you cannot synthesize yourself but without which you would stop replenishing your blood and producing new tissue for your muscles, skin, memory and so on. In short, you are keeping yourself alive. A genuine need is therefore one that provides us with the means of staying alive without us having to understand or justify it. You eat because you are hungry, you derive some pleasure from it and you keep on living. Here is another example. Sexual desire attracts you to the skin and smell of the person you desire. This desire leads to the meeting of bodies and inevitably to the reproduction of the species. Wherever the individual or the group has to survive, these natural impulses, these genuine needs, are at work. They are natural because they are part of our make-up, as much as our need to breathe. We are programmed to fulfil them and be rewarded in doing so.

But this is not all. The amazing pleasure of being rewarded is only the visible tip of the iceberg. The really important processes are taking place deep below in the depths.

When you have satisfied a 'genuine' need, you are rewarded with a pleasure that is deep, long lasting and free. These are the three criteria that distinguish genuine needs.

At the same time as the pleasure you feel, a 'thing' is spreading through you that you do not feel but which is vitally important. This inconspicuous flow, an invisible and primordial message whose extraordinary role I am going to tell you about, had no name. I have called it 'bene-satisfaction' since it is about both benefit and satisfaction.

The primitive centre in the brain responsible for our instinctive life and for protecting it is called the hypothalamus, which appeared with the first reptiles. The hypothalamus houses a sort of pulsating heart whose role is nothing less than to send out life! It fills reptiles, mammals, monkeys as well as humans with the desire to live. This pulsating life force, similar to a heartbeat, starts radiating out during the embryo's first few weeks of life and it carries on until death. This tells us the extent to which pleasure – and all it conceals and harbours – is the prime and sole driving force for both human and animal life.

I have taken this very long detour in order to explain to you that if you are overweight and suffering then this is because you have eaten over and above your biological needs, knowing full well that you were likely to put on weight. If you have done this over and over again, you did so because you needed to. This need was not a need for nutrition; it could only have been a need for pleasure. And without you really realizing it, this need for pleasure shows that you were not getting enough. You were not reaping sufficient pleasure. And given that pleasures are interchangeable, you gave in and went for the easiest one, the most immediate, most primeval, most animal pleasure, the one that has become deeply rooted inside us since the time of our first ancestors and whose emotive power is the most violent – the pleasure of eating.

I can only conclude that if you want to lose weight and remain slim you will only manage this by controlling your sources of pleasure and by looking after this wonderful 'bene-satisfaction'. And oat bran, in addition to all its metabolic and medicinal effects, can generate pleasure, an immediate 'hit' of sweetness, creaminess and emotion, while at the same time giving you the pleasure of seeing your pounds drop off. The pleasure of realizing yourself, and from the way others see you too, that at last you love yourself.

Some further vitally important information about pleasure. If you are trying to lose weight it will help you to understand what pleasure really is, the point of pleasure, how it is produced and, most importantly, how to use it when venturing through the bleak realm of displeasure and adversity.

Throughout my medical career, one of the most important and surprising things I have learnt from working with patients burdened with chronic weight problems is the importance of the emotional, emotive aspect of their relationship with their weight, their body image and their food. And even more so the importance of pleasure associated with every stage of their journey.

The big mistake, the tragic error of those who have overseen the struggle against weight problems, is that they have neglected or overlooked this aspect, sticking instead to logical, rational equations with numbers, calculations for working out surplus calories and surplus pounds, calories consumed and calories burnt up.

Generations of nutritionists and dieticians think that putting on weight was and still is caused by eating too many calories. So to lose weight all you need to do is reverse the balance that is in credit to one that is in debit, just as you would do with a business. Their reasoning is apparently watertight: eat less, exercise more and soon you will be back down to a normal weight. A watertight argument if it were intended for a robot or a baby being fed by some automatic wet nurse, but when intended for human beings, it is wrong from start to finish. To be sure, we human beings are rational but we are also prey to our emotions, our feelings, our joys, our sorrows, to our animal side and to our crucial need for pleasure in order to embrace life.

This energy consumption approach to weight problems and our relationship to food displays an immense lack of understanding of the forces we are dealing with here, of the very forces that create these weight problems.

Men and women who put on weight never do so without realizing what they are doing, by inadvertently eating the wrong foods or through careless mistakes that only need to be put right for those pounds accidentally gained to be lost again. My female patients, whom I systematically question on this point, tell me quite plainly, 'I eat badly, I eat too much, I eat everything I shouldn't eat.' They all know perfectly well that their eating lapses and binges, and repeatedly lapsing and bingeing, will make them fat. They hate this prospect, they hate themselves for doing it, they feel terribly guilty about it, they do it unwillingly and with the very greatest reluctance – but they still do it!

So why do they do it?

They are not looking for nutrients and even less so calories – it is pleasure they are after, driven by the most primeval centres in our instinctive and emotional brain. We share these centres with all other mammals; they are responsible for ensuring our immediate survival and they drown out any voice of reason.

In a painful world that is out of tune, in an environment where we feel stressed, under pressure and our quality of life and sources of pleasure are limited, the absolute imperative is to seek out some pleasure and gratification and urgently!

A woman living a hectic life, juggling her demanding career with children who take up much of her time and a home with all its many responsibilities, goes from one day to the next without getting enough pleasure. When this woman is then confronted with some greater than average stress, such as an emotional setback, hassle at work, too much work, anxiety, insomnia, her children having problems at school and so on, she is no longer in any position to listen to common-sense arguments reciting the virtues of a balanced diet: 'Eat less, exercise more!'

You do not teach a drowning person how to swim. Unfortunately there are some psychiatrists who still suggest this, oblivious of the harm they could be causing.

This drowning woman does not want to hear instructions in her day-to-day life about how she should endeavour to eat only when she feels natural, animal hunger pangs and then stop once they are satisfied.

What this woman wants is a quick fix of pleasure, sensual pleasure, relief, gratification; she wants to feel full, replenished and have her suffering and discomfort mopped up; she wants a crutch to keep herself upright.

So she eats.

Then she puts on weight.

However, the day comes when she has piled on so much weight that comfort foods are no longer enough to neutralize the stresses of everyday life and the torment of being overweight. If in such a situation there is some slight improvement, an upturn, a reason to feel more relaxed about her daily life – a child passing their exams, a promotion at work, she meets someone, anything warm and rewarding – then the pointer on the Pleasure/Displeasure scales moves to the other side and this ACTIVATES THE CHANGE. It triggers the longing and the resolve to make changes, to get back her old body, her old self-image, her confidence, her self-esteem – a determination to get out of the quagmire, a desire to lose weight and the sudden, brute strength to turn the vicious circle into a virtuous one and . . . **to find pleasure in doing this.**

Women who can feel this new life force rise up inside them know instinctively or from experience that this new strength flowing through them is as powerful as it is short-lived and that they must make the most of it as quickly as possible. What they then need and look for is a way of losing weight rapidly and of achieving tangible, encouraging results straightaway before the enthusiasm of this burst of motivation fades away.

The struggle that begins at this point revolves entirely around controlling pleasure. The woman who has become overweight has become so because of an irrepressible need to find pleasure or neutralize displeasure. By making up her mind to lose weight, not only will she have to cut off this source of compensatory pleasure but she will have to GO IN THE OPPOSITE DIRECTION, change over to a life of restrictions and move into a realm of frustration and displeasure.

To make this turnaround possible, she needs another source of satisfaction to replace the one she is giving up.

And she will find this pleasure in what is one of the most vital sources of nourishment for the individual – the EGO. By SUCCEEDING in losing weight, seeing SUCCESSFUL results at long last displayed on her bathroom scales, she will feel much better about herself.

Perhaps you are having trouble understanding how this substitution works, how pleasure from chocolate or cheese can be replaced by pleasure from managing to lose weight? Well, I quite understand why you are surprised.

Follow me carefully as there is a vitally important point here that is worth taking some time to explain.

When you travel to a country where a different currency is used, you change your money into this local currency, into dollars for example if you were in New York. What do these two currencies that you are converting one into the other have in common? A real shared value that allows you to obtain the exact same thing using both.

The same is true of pleasure, whose end purpose is to reward behaviour that promotes survival. In turn, the pleasure we feel fuels our need and our urge to live. Of all our needs this is the prime one, our subconscious clinging on to life.

This pleasure, like a currency, may appear in very different forms that have no apparent connection. Sexual pleasure, parental pleasure, aesthetic pleasure, spiritual pleasure and pleasure from exercising power – all these pleasures convey a common nourishment which ends up on the same receptors in our ancient brains and, as the saying goes, 'never mind the bottle, let's just drink what's inside!' Never mind what the pleasure is, as long as it travels from transmitter substance to transmitter substance, endorphins, serotonin, dopamine, until it reaches that part of our brain that sends out the motivation to live.

However, each and every one of us, due to our nature or our nurture, is attracted to one or more of these pleasures and has a natural ability to grasp them.

A woman who agrees to do without comfort food as her crutch absolutely MUST find another support. Any sensible weight-loss programme that wants to get results must make it possible for her to find compensation elsewhere. Pleasure from eating must become less of an obsession as the slimmer learns to find gratification from a different source of satisfaction.

What other sources are there?

There are four measures that allow slimmers to bring some pleasure back into their lives while dieting:

1.   A diet that gets off to a quick and sure start
Pleasure from and enthusiasm for a diet that works. Short-term, heavy restrictions you can stick to while still 'anaesthetized' by the initial results you are achieving at remarkable speed. A diet that is the very opposite of those that drag on and on, that sow doubt and weaken resolve. This is why my programme starts with a short Attack phase lasting two to seven days, depending on how much you are aiming to lose; short but with rapid results – on average, a couple of pounds by the end of the first three days or twice as much after six. And our precious oat bran galette boosts these results, both by sneaking away calories and filling up the stomach.

2. A hunger-free diet

The pleasure of not feeling hungry when on a diet is a powerful impetus.

Hunger from cutting back on quantities heralds disaster for a diet in the short, medium and long term. The doctor or adviser responsible for prescribing 120g (4oz) fish with 100g (3½oz) rice, 25g (1oz) cheese and one square of chocolate for an evening meal is once again going back to what all the text books on nutrition have been teaching for the past 60 years. Unfortunately by doing this, however noble the doctor's intentions, they demonstrate their profound lack of understanding about how a fat person's mind works.

A weary woman at her wit's end, who when she arrives home after an hour on public transport agrees not to raid her fridge but instead get her kids ready for bed, who is then faced with a menu like the one above is, despite all her good intentions, hardly likely to emerge unscathed.

One square of chocolate! I can hear one of my patients sharing with me what she thought about one of the last diets she had been shackled to: 'One square of chocolate – once a bar of chocolate is opened it sends out strong signals that only stop once it's finished! I am one of those people, doctor, who can't do anything by halves. I go to extremes and I'm only comfortable if it's all or nothing.' This is why my method is based on a very simple premise – you are free to eat the foods you are allowed but you forget about everything else for a short but strict period: 100 foods, 72 from animals, 28 from vegetables. You can eat AS MUCH AS YOU WANT of them all. This includes oat bran, which swells up in the stomach, speedily encouraging satisfaction and satiety.

3. A diet with a strong support structure

The pleasure from having a strong, reassuring framework means you can tolerate many restrictions. This framework, the diet's structure, is its internal organization, the way in which it has been put together so that dieters can lean on it as they follow its key guidelines.

This idea of structure may appear abstract but in fact it is of paramount importance. What troubles overweight people who feel tempted to try and lose weight is not knowing where to start and what to do. What foods should you stick to? Should you drink a lot or not? Do you count calories or work with different food groups? And even those who know what to do need someone to give them the starting signal. Surprising as it may seem, this is how it is. All recent studies on behavioural psychology have proven how important an outside authority is for instructions to be carried out.

I have concluded from a lifetime of direct experience of diets and monitoring them that the way the instructions are set up, a way that is directive and completely interconnected, is at least as important as the actual instructions themselves.

By definition, any diet stops you from eating what you want. De facto it leads to restriction and frustration. What is actually most difficult about dieting is forcing yourself to make unappealing decisions. It is infinitely less frustrating and easier to follow clear-cut instructions if an external agent provides them and if there is no hope of negotiation.

I developed my programme in the light of such evidence and its instructions are clear, precise, concrete and unambiguous.

You can eat what you want of the foods that are allowed; any other foods, for a clearly defined period, are to be left well alone.

My method comprises four completely interconnected phases with a programme that leaves nothing to chance:

- A short, productive Attack phase with lightning-quick results, tailored to every kind of case.
- A Cruise phase that takes you straight to your True Weight, at an average speed of a couple of pounds a week.
- A Consolidation phase that lasts five days for every pound lost, with its two portions of starchy foods and two celebration meals a week.
- A permanent Stabilization phase with its famous protein Thursdays, giving up lifts and escalators and 20 minutes' walking every day, and three tablespoonfuls of oat bran a day FOR LIFE.

4. PLEASURE factored in as an antidote to restriction
However complicated life may be, the appeal of pleasure and repulsion of displeasure are always being weighed

up. At every moment, without you even being aware of it, a compass in your brain is calculating the cost of even the least activity you may have to get involved in. If I do this what pleasure would I get from it? Would it not be better to do this instead, as it will bring me just as much pleasure but sooner? Perhaps, but doing that would have troublesome, frustrating, even painful repercussions which would scupper that choice...

From the brain's anatomy and cerebral imaging we have managed to discover an extraordinarily important fact: there are links connecting the centres of pleasure with the centres of displeasure; pleasure is able to inhibit displeasure. This means nothing less than: USING PLEASURE CAN REDUCE SUFFERING. You will understand this better if I draw a parallel that in practice you all know about. When you are overcome by stress, you feel like putting food that is more comforting and scrumptious than usual into your mouth, to make contact with your taste buds and then slip down your pharynx; you stuff yourself with it to make yourself feel good. It is a little like going into a room heated by a radiator in the middle of winter when you are freezing cold – I know precisely the direction in which your pleasure brain would take you!

Putting on weight means you are eating more than you need nutritionally, but you create pleasure. Losing weight means taking the opposite path – it means putting up with frustration to lose those surplus pounds.

It is possible, it is even essential, to make every endeavour to sublimate what is allowed in a diet, so that it becomes cloaked in pleasure. Is there anything more raw and rustic than a freshly felled pine tree? What could be more inviting, more symbolic and more thrilling than a Christmas tree? It only takes a few tree lights, baubles and some tinsel. My Dukan Diet recipes must become the tree lights, baubles and tinsel that keep you on track with your diet. The 350 recipes in *The Dukan Diet Recipe Book* and *The Complete Dukan Cookbook* are a fantastic source of expertise and knowledge, and they have come from those who, after my family, are dearest to me – my patients, my readers and my diet's enthusiastic fans, who over the years have shown me so much affection. This little treasure trove must be used as a pleasure generator, practical proof of what I am advocating: the art of braving displeasure's chill winds by finding pleasure and creating warmth.

When my daughter Maya pointed me towards oat bran, little did she know that she was entrusting me with a secret that thousands of other women would go on to share. In my long career spent helping others tackle the agonies of being overweight I have seen all the discomfort, insecurity, anguish, stress and suffering involved. Putting on weight does harm and losing weight does good. That is the reason why I have worked for so many years to do all I can to help my patients lose weight, because knowing their joy I was able to feed from their pleasure and their self-fulfilment – pure selfishness on my part!

In conclusion, returning to oat bran and the three kinds of pleasure it can provide:

- My diet works better when oat bran is part of it and the pleasure gained from losing weight is increased. My statistics, comparing results before and after oat bran was included in my diet, clearly establish that the method works better with it: you lose weight more effectively, more rapidly and with a greater likelihood of stabilizing.
- Quite simply, oat bran tastes good and because of this it produces pleasure. You can make dishes and recipes with very enjoyable slow sugars using oat bran without fearing any drawbacks as regards metabolism or calories.
- Oat bran curbs the appetite and makes us feel full quicker. My diet had no restrictions on certain high-protein foods and vegetables and by including oat bran it now offers the luxurious pleasure of losing weight with no fear of going hungry.

How much oat bran can you use and when?

It could not be easier to use.

- If you are in my Attack phase, which lasts two to seven days depending on your circumstances, age, weight history, how long you have been overweight, the number of diets you have tried and whether or not you need to get off to rapid start, you are allowed one and a half heaped tablespoonfuls of oat bran.
- In the Cruise phase, you can increase this to two tablespoonfuls.
- In the Consolidation phase, you can go up to three.
- In permanent Stabilization, you MUST take three.

As for how you use it, that is up to you and you will find lots of recipes at the end of the book.

How oat bran is manufactured and what makes it effective

Be aware that there are different types of oat bran – depending on how they are milled and sifted – and they are not all of equal merit. Oat bran's medicinal benefits, both for helping with weight problems as well as cholesterol and slowing down sugar assimilation depend on two production variables – how the bran is milled and how it is sifted.

Milling

The extent to which the bran is milled defines the size of the oat bran particle. There are three main milling grades: coarse, medium and fine. Each of these three milling grades is then sub-divided into either a simple or a 'bis' process, so in all there are six milling grades that produce six different particle sizes. The size of the particle produced by the milling process will determine the flavour and texture of the bran when we eat it, how long it can be cooked and of course its physical properties too; how much it can absorb and its viscosity, which are both responsible for it medicinal effects.

If the milling is too fine, the plant texture and oat bran fibre are damaged. This sort of milling turns the bran into powdery flour that is great to cook with and for making cakes, desserts, muffins, bread and pizza bases. However, if milled finely, the bran can no longer absorb very much, has less surface viscosity and so it is far less medicinal.

Likewise if the bran is not milled enough and is too coarse, it becomes rough and very difficult to eat and it also loses that useful surface viscosity.

Sifting

Sifting is the process whereby the milled oat bran is sifted to separate the actual grain, full of fast-release carbohydrates, and the outer husk which contains very little carbohydrate but is packed with betaglucan molecules, the medicinal active agent in bran. So it follows that the more the bran is sifted, the purer it becomes, the more betaglucans it contains and it will be more effective. Bran than has not been sufficiently sifted will contain too many fast sugars. Such bran is sweeter and tastes nicer but is far less useful if you are trying to get your weight down.

Cooking bran and medicinal bran

Research on the impact that oat bran has on weight loss, cholesterol, glycaemic index and digestion shows that the quality of the results depends on the size and purity of the bran particle, i.e. on getting the optimum milling and sifting combination

We see that there are two different types of oat bran depending on how it is produced; cooking bran that is very fine and sifted only a little, and medicinal bran produced by intermediate milling with sifting that really separates the husks from the grains.

From studies that have been carried out, it has been

possible to work out what effects the different types of oat bran have by testing the different products produced by the different manufacturing processes. Criteria for how effective the various brans are medicinally, based on the various milling and sifting combinations, are monitored from functional coprology and nutritional residue recovered from stools. As you have read, oat bran works medicinally by slowing down digestion and assimilating fats and carbohydrates in the intestinal bolus and in so doing it ends up reducing the number of calories ingested.

Optimum milling is Medium Bis, M2bis, which produces a particle slightly broader than the standard medium size.

Optimum sifting is B6, here the bran is sifted six times which ensures that it only contains a negligible amount of fast carbohydrates.

Together both indexes make up an overall M2bis-B6 index.

Most manufacturers, particularly those in Anglo-Saxon countries, sell bran only for its culinary qualities; they favour very fine milling and superficial sifting, producing bran that is sweet and chewy to eat but not really suitable for medicinal purposes.

Recent studies and research have compared and contrasted oat bran's culinary and medicinal qualities. It is important that international producers, manufacturers and retailers change the way they manufacture oat bran so that everyone can buy bran with all these many invaluable medicinal properties.

Although of course the cost of producing medicinal oat bran compared with bran purely for culinary purposes is a little higher, the nutritional benefits are far greater.

Part II:

A health food

Oat bran, the heart and cholesterol

- Of known natural foods, oat bran is the one that most effectively lowers cholesterol levels.
- It is the only foodstuff in America that is allowed to claim 'good for the heart' on its packaging.
- It is the first foodstuff to be given 'nutraceutical' status by the American Food and Drug Administration, well known for its strict criteria.

I have headed this chapter with these three statements to focus your attention on oat bran's amazing properties.

I would like to point out in passing that however beneficial this foodstuff may be, it is not easy to buy. Do you know why this is so?

Because it is too cheap! It is inexpensive and takes up too much space in a shop display. A packet of oat bran costs only a pound or two and competes for space that 15 or 20 packs of food supplements could fill. Nobody is interested in marketing it, yet in actual fact it is such an invaluable and health-protecting foodstuff that it ought to be available on the National Health Service.

So I say once again, if I have taken the time to write a book about the beneficial effects of this modest cereal, it is because simply looking at the incidence of heart problems and diabetes in rich nations and considering all that oat bran can do, I estimate that it could help prevent half the deaths.

Let us turn our attention to cholesterol – you have no

doubt heard about this substance that clogs up our arteries. You may also have read a lot about the cholesterol content of certain foods. Such familiarity should in no way trivialize its role and its dangers.

Nowadays in the Western world high cholesterol is a real public enemy, responsible for almost half the deaths. If we eliminate secondary causes to illustrate the point, overall you stand a 50 per cent chance of dying from heart disease and a 50 per cent chance of dying from cancer. And with heart-related diseases, cholesterol always plays a fatal role.

I want to make it clear that I am not drawing your attention to some minor or occasional danger. In order to reassure themselves, some people still think that high cholesterol is only a problem that concerns the elderly. Yet young people are equally affected by it. Cholesterol blocks the arteries, and as for which ones are most affected, unfortunately it is the coronary arteries that take the prize. Sadly we hear a lot about these arteries getting blocked as this causes infarction and angina pectoris; in addition, blocked arteries in the brain lead to strokes.

Regardless of your gender and your age, you can be sure that a little cholesterol has already been deposited in your arteries, just as you have tartar deposits on your teeth. This silent, unassuming killer, camouflaged behind such commonplace foods as an omelette, entrecote steak or a piece of Cheddar, targets each and every one of us.

From the age of 20, it is a good idea to be routinely tested for cholesterol levels every five years, as there is nothing worse than it building up over time without you knowing it. From the age of 45 onwards, it is wise to have an annual test, especially if recent results are over the limit.

Lastly, since we are tracking down the most effective serial killer in Western history you ought to know a little more about this disturbing character. When we mention cholesterol without any further qualification, we are talking about 'total' cholesterol, which includes 'bad' cholesterol but 'good' cholesterol too.

Bad cholesterol is the viscous sort, the one that sticks and clogs up arteries. Every time the heart pumps blood, which leaves from the aorta and returns via the pulmonary artery, a tiny quantity of cholesterol gets deposited.

It is you, your liver, that produces this bad cholesterol from animal fats. From the fats in the animals that we breed, that we keep in pens and fatten up before we kill them. By poisoning us *post mortem*, they are taking their revenge.

Good cholesterol is the very opposite and is both the antidote for bad cholesterol and its foe. It works just like a detergent – detergents lift away fats.

In a nutshell, bad cholesterol clogs up your arteries and good cholesterol unclogs them. If you are fortunate enough to produce good cholesterol you can tolerate much higher levels of total cholesterol. To increase the amount of good cholesterol in your blood you need to:

- Eat fish
- Take exercise
- Drink one to two glasses of wine a day
- And, most importantly of all, give up smoking

Those are the main facts you need to know about cholesterol.

If, like most people, you work hard in life to better yourself, to achieve the goals that you deem extremely important, for example a qualification or a promotion, then allow me to tell you about oat bran and how it can help you accomplish so much more.

Cholesterol is mostly produced in the liver. It then travels along the bile ducts to the intestines. Like all fatty bodies it enters the bloodstream and there it flows round and round, leaving the heart only to return there, day and night, throughout your life.

Let's take a closer look at this cholesterol as it passes through the small intestine. Here it gets mixed in with the pulped nutrients, the food bolus that is the end product after your food has been chemically processed.

If you eat oat bran regularly, your intestinal bolus will be full of bran and as the cholesterol comes into contact with its soluble fibre it behaves just as it does on the walls of your arteries. The cholesterol gets into the fibre, sticks to it and seeps into the fibre's microscopic vacuoles.

Since this catch-all fibre cannot be absorbed by the human body, it passes right through the small intestine, then through the large colon, ending up in our stools, taking with it the bit of cholesterol that withstood being absorbed by the blood and its powerful sucking.

It is estimated that if enough oat bran is eaten regularly, blood cholesterol from food may be lowered by 15 per cent. This is equivalent to results obtained by taking some of the main medication for hypercholesterolaemia (high cholesterol).

Do bear in mind that although oat bran has been proven to lower cholesterol, it may not always reduce it sufficiently, especially if the cholesterol is well established and the levels are already high. The threat is greater if the deposits are long-standing and have never been treated. If you have been prescribed statins or fibrates, do not cut them down without your doctor's permission.

However, for anyone with a cholesterol level that is close to becoming a pathology, oat bran is a genuine solution and particularly so when used by young people. It is rare for a predisposition to high cholesterol not to worsen over time, and time is precious as the deposits will keep building up.

Oat bran should also be recommended to anyone who still has normal levels but where there is a family history of high cholesterol or of cardiac or cardiovascular problems.

You will have grasped that oat bran is as much a cure as it is a prevention. If you are predisposed to high cholesterol and to being overweight, the benefits of eating oat bran will be twofold for you.

So look upon this humble cereal as a friend that has

your best interests at heart. And, I am choosing my words carefully here, a friend that may even save your life. So eat it any way you like – in milk, yoghurt or fromage frais. Make galettes, pancakes and blinis with it.

Learn to enjoy this bran day after day. Become a devotee because if you are predisposed to cholesterol or weight problems, they will never leave you in peace.

If you want to make the bran work even more effectively, try adding some linseed or sesame seeds to your blinis and enjoying them with a nice slice of smoked salmon or sardine fillet in olive oil. The effects of the bran will be boosted by the linolenic acid in the sesame seeds, the deep sea fish oils and the beneficial properties of the olive oil.

Oat bran and diabetes

As with weight problems and cholesterol, oat bran works in another remarkable way: it combats diabetes by slowing down the rate at which the body absorbs sugars.

Being extremely soluble, oat bran fibre can, when combined with fast sugars, slow down the rate at which they pass through the digestive tract and enter the bloodstream.

As soon as the oat bran is in your mouth and becomes soaked with saliva, this slowing down starts. Then comes the slow journey through the stomach until it reaches the small intestine, a crucial place since it is here that the food, now broken down into its basic components, can be absorbed. Once it reaches the small intestine, the bran once again acts as a screen between the intestinal bolus and the walls of the small intestine.

Let us take a look now at why this property that oat bran has turns out to be so invaluable for diabetics.

In our collective subconscious, we see diabetes as historically a worrying disease but fortunately confined to moribund old people. Of course, viewing diabetes this way is ridiculous as it can hit people at any age. All the same, diabetes is a condition that does take time to develop. However, this being so, we tend only to react to this dangerously silent illness once the harm has been done and a diagnosis is given.

Tucked away in the middle of your abdomen, you have

an organ called the pancreas which is involved in the digestive process. But what concerns us here is that it is the pancreas that secretes insulin, a key hormone in our human physiology. When you have a meal, you eat foods that are bound to contain a sizeable portion of carbohydrates, our main source of fuel, of which there are three separate sub-families. They differ from one another in the way that their basic elements are assembled, so consequently our bodies absorb them at different rates and speeds.

The first family is slow sugars and we call them complex carbohydrates. Because they are made up of chains of molecules that are so long and so fused together that they can only be broken down into their basic elements over time, they get absorbed gradually and slowly. You will know them by the common but inappropriate name of starches or starchy foods, a term which through use has ended up being adopted. This family includes cereals – wheat, rice, corn, rye, oats and so on. It also includes tubers, potatoes being the most common example. Finally there are legumes lentils, beans, all kinds of peas, etc.

A second family of less complex sugars includes fructose, the sugar in fruit; it takes less to break it down so it enters the bloodstream more rapidly and easily. When consumed in its natural form as pieces of fruit and not as fruit juice, the fibre in the skin and fruit pulp slows this process down slightly. Milk provides lactose, a sugar with a similar structure which gets absorbed a little more slowly.

The third family, simple sugars and sugary products – of which classic white table sugar is the most common and widely used example – have molecules that are assembled and structured far more easily.

Over the past 50 years, consumption of this industrially processed sugar has steadily risen in all Western countries, whereas consumption of bread and vegetables has declined. Demand for sugar has increased in every sector of food retailing. Why is this so?

There are two reasons. Firstly, it is the only nutrient there is that has a sweet taste, a flavour that we are instinctively drawn towards, and this attraction is further reinforced by the messages we see around us. Another reason is that it can be quickly absorbed. Eating a high-sugar product gives us instant pleasure in our mouths and an immediate feeling of satisfaction as the sugar works subtly on certain transmitter substances such as serotonin, more widely known as the happiness hormone. It is easy to understand why sugar is the most common comfort food as it gives us quick, intense pleasure – a 'high'. And pleasure means 'bene-satisfaction' and producing chemicals in our brain that satisfy and maintain our lust for life.

In other words, pleasure and getting pleasure over and over again in our daily lives is very closely connected with our life energy. It would therefore be unthinkable and even dangerous to try and tame or lessen our need for such small daily pleasures.

In this family of rapid sugars, you will recognize

sweets, pastries, biscuits and everything we tend to describe with the ambiguous and revealing term 'sweet things'. The simple sugar that we most quickly absorb is glucose, which enters our bloodstream 'as if it were completely at home' and with good reason – it is our own natural fuel and the one we test for when checking our blood sugar levels.

These then are the three families of sugars that make up the wide category of carbohydrates. They each have their own particular taste, consistency and appearance. However, once digested they end up being reduced to identical basic elements. They all finish up in our bloodstream but, because how they withstand being broken down differs, how they come into contact with the wall of the small intestine will vary widely too. Blood glucose levels – glycaemia – go up more or less abruptly depending on the sugar type and which foods are providing them. How high the blood sugar level rises depends on how quickly these sugars travel through the digestive tract and, most importantly, how well they are absorbed.

This is where insulin gets involved.

When a meal is packed with carbohydrates, especially the sort that are massively and quickly absorbed, our blood sugar level suddenly shoots up. Our bodies have difficulty tolerating this excess glucose circulating in the blood as it ends up becoming toxic. This toxicity is all the more dangerous as the blood's job is to carry glucose, energy and oxygen to every part of the body, so no organ is spared the effects of this sugar-packed blood.

As soon as our blood sugar level rises above 1g per litre, the body reacts and the pancreas secretes insulin. The hormone's job is to drive the glucose in the blood-stream back to the two places where it is stored naturally, the liver and muscles.

The liver stores it away as glycogen, readily available to meet the needs of the individual, depending on levels of consumption and activity, so that any interruptions in supply are avoided.

As for our muscles, they are the main organs in the body to use glucose and they can store enough to cover their on-going energy requirements.

Things work differently for diabetics. A diabetic's pancreas is genetically fragile and vulnerable. Glucose intolerant, the pancreas overreacts when glucose enters the bloodstream by secreting too much insulin, too suddenly, and this tires it out. With time, and a diet containing too much sugar, the only outcome for a pancreas that is made to work as often and as hard as this is to become worn out.

In times of food shortages, when people ate frugally and had a low life expectancy, it was rare for a weakened pancreas to have the time and opportunity to show any signs of its fragility or of the complications caused by this fragility.

Statistically, the onset of Type 2 diabetes is around the age of 50 when the pancreas starts to malfunction. If not treated, major complications will arise in the next five years. Since for a long time life expectancy did not exceed

55, morbidity and mortality caused by diabetes did not cause much alarm.

Nowadays, the situation for diabetics is quite different and much more threatening. Fast-sugar consumption has literally exploded, physical activity has been practically eradicated and over the past century life expectancy has almost doubled.

To meet production demands, and in an attempt to attract as many consumers as possible with a seductive offer, the food-processing industry has capitalized on the wide range of sweet flavours available by using them as a marketing tool to create products that are ever more gratifying, seductive and appealing to our senses. The campaign to win over the general public starts early on, with children, who are still very much in touch with their genetic sugar dependence. Since the 1960s, new products have appeared every year that make ever greater use of fast sugars, refined cereals and processed milk, for example in white bread, pastries, sweets, confectionery, milky puddings and ice creams, not to mention the never-ending array of fizzy drinks and breakfast cereals. These are all launched amid much publicity and advertising that emphasizes the link between sugar and pleasure, sugar and well-being and sugar and reward.

When we get this combination of food abundance, a sedentary lifestyle and a body under strain, then genetic weaknesses start to become apparent.

When considering the ways in which oat bran can help prevent disease, you must keep in mind that having a fragile pancreas and being predisposed to diabetes is something that runs in families and is passed on through the genes. This means that there are families of diabetics, and it is these same families that from the earliest age need to take steps to protect their health and prevent illness. Even if there is only a *likelihood* of a condition being passed on – as with eye colour, it is always possible that a child will take after the parent who is not affected – preventive measures are necessary. They have to be presented and explained in a way that is flexible and not-too-restrictive over the long term, if only to lighten the pancreas' load. The earlier preventive measures are put in place, the better they will work. It is even possible to live your whole life without this illness developing.

There are two main ways of taking preventive measures.

First and foremost, by limiting the use of fast sugars and sweet-tasting foods, and treating them instead as reward-foods that diabetics must only ever eat occasionally.

There is absolutely no question of banning them and less so of demonizing them; however, controlling their consumption is important.

Obviously if you are simply getting a child or teenager to take *preventive* action, they have to be allowed some freedom to eat the foods that are popular among their age group. What is important, though, is that they understand that this freedom needs to be monitored and, most importantly, the reason why this is so. The best explanation is the parent who has diabetes.

Today, the human diet has become 'diabetogenous'. Not only have we got used to eating extreme flavours but competition between the big food-processing companies has led them to exploit sweetness as a marketing tool, just as they do with salts, fats, colouring and attractive packaging. No thought has been given to what the repercussions might be on the individuals of a species which is not just unprepared for this onslaught but, quite the opposite, is programmed not to be able to survive it.

Educating ourselves to limit our fast-sugar intake must be counterbalanced by some freedom to eat slow sugars, which the vast majority of children and teenagers are firmly attached to. There is an excellent opportunity here for parents to pass on the correct message about the differences between the many members of the carbohydrate family.

It is important to get the younger generation to understand what happens to the food they put in their mouths, digest and allow inside their final sanctuary, namely their own blood. Likewise it is worthwhile explaining to them how their bodies use these various sugars, which behave as differently inside our body's engine as different types of petrol, unleaded and diesel, do inside a combustion engine.

Children and teenagers are not as resistant to the idea of eating healthily as people like to think. On numerous occasions I have given talks to sixth formers and students of all levels, and I have been struck by how interested they are in what they eat.

I remember once going to talk to a final year class when the head teacher had expressed doubts about how much interest the class would show. Finding the pupils quite unsettled, I started off by asking them to put their hand up if they had a relative with diabetes then to do the same if their mum or dad had had stroke, heart or cardiovascular problems, and finally if someone close to them had had cancer.

In a trice, almost half these teenagers had their hand in the air. They were rapt with attention. My aim was to make them aware of ways in which they could protect themselves from the risks running in their family by eating correctly. I can assure you they did pay attention and they were interested. As chance would have it, there was a teenager with diabetes in this class, and a few others whose parents had had a rough time because their pathology had not been detected early enough. I honestly believe that preventive measures will only work if we appeal to instinct and emotion. These must prevail over rationality and overly abstract, scholarly demonstrations.

Promoting exercise is the second way to prevent illness.

Here again, this idea must not be put across in a scholarly, mandatory way. Instead it needs to be explained that using our bodies will greatly improve muscle tone as well as how they work and look.

Diabetics have to be made to understand that their muscles have lost the ability to store excess blood sugar which is why their glycaemic level goes up until it becomes toxic. To enable the muscles to regain this ability, a diabetic has to work them regularly. An example that always hits home is that, when properly worked, a muscle will burn up far more calories than you might imagine – on average 30 minutes of brisk walking burns up 144 calories, 30 minutes of rollerskating 216 calories, 30 minutes of cycling 340 calories and, if you can face walking up stairs for 30 minutes, this burns up 460 calories! But do you know what happens when you stop exercising? The muscle keeps working for 72 hours; at a lower rate, to be sure, but for every hour of the day, day and night, and even when you are asleep. And this work is proportionate to the size of the muscle. So it is absolutely vital to work your muscles both to lose weight and to develop your muscle mass.

These preventive measures must be taken seriously if the diabetic wants to avoid the nightmare of having to check on a regular basis that most of their organs are working properly. Those organs most at risk are the heart, eyes, kidneys and nervous system.

Oat bran reveals how incredibly effective it can be by again offering a way of preventing disease. How does it do this?

As soon as it is in the mouth, the bran forms a big gelatinous net with the food, infiltrating and sticking to the food as it is being ground up and liquefied. Already mixed in with the food, the bran forces it to pass through the stomach more slowly by delaying the opening of the pylorus. During this time the food and bran are subjected to mechanical churning and local acidity. The pylorus will only open once the stomach's contents are sufficiently fluid to flow out into the small intestine.

Once again it is here in the small intestine that oat bran's specific properties come into their own. The fast sugars, the first to arrive, will be immobilized and caught in the fine, sticky mesh of the bran's net.

When this happens, the blood, which is greedy for its sugar and is demanding its nutrient, sets off powerful suction within the small intestine so that most of these sugars end up being dislodged and sucked up but at a much slower rate than when there is no oat bran. A small amount of these sugars, too firmly entangled, will resist and, after a lengthy journey through the large intestine, they will end up in the stools with the fibre.

So oat bran not only delays the progress of sugars through the alimentary canal from one end to the other, so that they pass and get absorbed into the bloodstream over a longer period of time, but the bran actually gets rid of a modest but nonetheless appreciable amount of sugar.

As a result, having oat bran in the digestive system transforms fast sugars into slow sugars. This means it is possible to avoid massive glycaemic spikes that 'batter' the pancreas, forcing it to secrete huge quantities of insulin which eventually ends up wearing the pancreas out. What is more, it is worth being aware that as well as dealing directly and specifically with sugars, insulin also stimulates our appetite and encourages us to store away fat, so it makes us put on weight. Since being overweight paves the way for diabetes and exacerbates the condition, we find ourselves in a vicious circle that only leads to further diabetes and weight problems, with cardiovascular complications following in the wake of both.

Take careful note! Let there be no ambiguity here – oat bran's job is not to sort out the problem of diabetes all on its own. Once diabetes has been diagnosed there is nowadays a whole range of medication that, when taken in the right combination, can keep the blood sugar level below toxic concentrations. None of these medicines can cure diabetes but by using them in conjunction you can try and delay the development of the disease and, by so doing, delay complications from appearing too.

Prevention is the only really intelligent treatment. Precisely because it is still incurable, in families where there is a history of diabetes and a strong likelihood of the disease developing, everything hinges on eating correctly and taking exercise during the first half of a person's life, the period of latency when medication is of no use whatsoever. And on this battle front reserved for food, oat bran is a major ally.

The most crucial time to be using oat bran is when diabetes first starts to slowly take hold. In cases where there is a family history of diabetes and a blood test shows for the first time that the blood sugar level has reached and exceeded 1.10g per litre, and this level does not change over six months, oat bran can on its own delay the onset of this incipient disease. It can even hold it in check if everything is done to prevent the diabetes, and this includes taking exercise.

How much oat bran should be taken and when?

Take the maximum dose straightaway and in whatever way you want: in dairy products, pancakes, galettes, blinis, pizza bases etc., and take a minimum of three tablespoonfuls per day.

For optimum results, it is best to have one tablespoonful in the morning, two at lunchtime and two in the evening.

Ideally oat bran should be eaten as part of a meal so that it becomes thoroughly combined with your food. Once again, if you are taking it in pancakes, limit the number of whole eggs you consume to one a day.

Finally, as diabetes may occur alongside weight and cholesterol problems, using oat bran is strongly recommended for this very high risk combination.

To sum up, be vigilant. If you are young and you are not diabetic but one of your parents has the disease, look upon oat bran as your friend – I will never tire of saying this. If both your parents have diabetes then not eating oat bran is not only daft but it is a mistake.

It has now been proven that oat bran slows down the rate at which sugars pass through the digestive system. By including enough bran in your diet you have absolutely nothing to lose and everything to gain. If, early on, you start using it regularly, I am convinced you will live to a riper age and enjoy better health.

Oat bran and cancer

There are two ways in which oat bran can help prevent cancer. By helping to control weight problems, it helps prevent cancer of the colon.

Studies carried out and statistics collected from across the world show an unequivocal correlation between being overweight and getting cancer. Anything that can bring down obesity levels will help limit the overall incidence of cancer.

And because of the way oat bran works as a screen inside the body, like some other types of easily tolerated fibre, it protects us from cancers in the digestive system and, most especially, from cancer of the colon, one of the most common forms of the disease in humans.

Research undertaken in many international epidemiological studies has shown that in countries where the populations eat lots of cereals and, by extension, vegetable fibre, people suffer far less from cancer of the colon than in those countries where a more sophisticated food industry means the cereals consumed are processed and contain less fibre.

This is an appropriate moment to take a closer look at how food industry manufacturers, decision-makers in food retailing and admen influence the average consumer's dietary habits.

For these three groups, who control the food we are supplied with, who steer our needs and very often shape our desires and tastes, their business is to pursue two simple goals: to keep on producing more and more, and to find new consumers.

Our daily lives are moulded and structured by being consumers. For most of us in the West, our fundamental needs – that is, those ensuring our survival and reproduction, particularly having easy access to food – have been taken care of for over a century now. Hunger has been practically eradicated from our affluent countries.

On the other hand, many other needs which are connected not with our survival but rather with our quality of life, happiness and self-fulfilment have become very much more difficult to satisfy.

Our sexuality has become impoverished, as complementarity between the sexes has been lost.

The world of work has become tougher and more fragmented.

Our housing is valued according to the numbers of bedrooms, and the home is no longer the family's centre of gravity.

Belonging to the group has turned into mass slavery, a mass that is no longer made up of supportive and familiar individuals.

Machines have been allowed to dispossess us of our body's instinctive pleasure in doing things to live.

Our need for nature, the earth, the sea, the forests, a clear sky and animals is to a large extent no longer fulfilled.

Our need to play in order to develop as humans and learn about life has more often than not nowadays been reduced to living in the passive world of television.

The need for something sacred, a fundamental part of all past societies and civilizations, has forsaken ours, diminishing our destinies and the meaning of our lives.

And our need for something of beauty, so close to the sacred, has given way to the cult of the useful, to speculation, to the 'art market'!

All these needs and pleasures, which set humanity apart, are not individual or cultural conquests but are programmed in our genes. Today they have been supplanted by other needs, which are purely economic – society's needs. Nowadays, our lifestyle tends to thwart natural sources of satisfaction that cost nothing and replace them with superficial, artificial sources that are sold at a price.

As far as food is concerned, we could not have a more abundant offering. Our food is being constantly updated so that we never tire of it. Addiction tools make use of increasingly intense flavours that are similar to psychotropic substances, so powerful is their effect on our brains. Furthermore, these products are designed to look as magnetic, sexy and alluring as possible. Even many of our fruits and vegetables undergo extensive treatment to be smooth and shiny, graded and devoid of the slightest imperfection. If not, then nobody will be interested in them! 'Misshapen' vegetables, fruit with markings or of a colour that simply looks suspect to our sanitized minds and eyes – in other words, the very fruit and vegetables our ancestors happily ate – are automatically destroyed.

A health food

As smooth and artificial products gain the upper hand, anything that smacks of being natural or homely finds itself ghettoized and consigned to the 'organic' niche. We must have foodstuffs that taste domesticated, docile and undemanding.

This is why we now eat white bread, the rich man's bread. Farewell to the peasant's unrefined flour. Modern man has been trained to enjoy the rich man's city loaf, bread made from white flour, stripped of the texture of its natural fibre. The same is true of all starchy foods produced on an industrial scale – pasta, pre-cooked rice and freeze-dried potato products.

For a century now, to satisfy production demands, a little more use is being made each year of refined, nutritionally depleted, denatured foods, full of pesticides, colouring, additives, texturizing agents and flavour enhancers. We end up then with products that have no texture or natural waste but are packed with all sorts of chemicals and allergens that pollute our digestive systems. Overrefined products build up in the colon and bowel movements start to become less regular. Matter and waste stagnate and at the same time the dangerous products they are carrying around start to accumulate and spend more time in contact with the intestinal wall. Among these products are some that are actually carcinogenic.

What might have seemed to you to be a digression is unfortunately the most serious reason put forward today to explain why cancer of the colon keeps on steadily increasing.

At the same time, a lot of studies seem to provide proof that being overweight or obese creates a carcinogenic effect, especially among women. Adipocytes – the cells involved in storing fat – have an oestrogenic hormonal action that we know can be badly tolerated by the tissue in female sex organs, the womb and breasts. In the case of people who, to put it bluntly, are overweight and in particular obese, once their adipocytes have become enlarged and can no longer hold any extra fat, the cells divide. Obese people not only have more fat but also more adipocytes and therefore more oestrogen, and so are at greater risk of getting women's cancers. All cancer specialists know this and insist that any patients at risk need to tackle their weight and stop being obese.

Oat bran protects against cancer in two ways. It works inside the body to protect the mucous membrane in the colon and, more generally, it helps reduce weight and thus limit the impact on our hormones of being overweight.

Oat bran acts against weight problems on several fronts and in different ways. Let us recap:

- Oat bran is filling.
- It has a pleasant taste and texture.
- It contains a lot of proteins.
- Producing insulin encourages us to store fat and oat bran reduces insulin production.
- And, most importantly, oat bran sneaks away calories in the small intestine as it takes hold of nutrients and calories, dragging them away in the stools.

All these properties put together allow us to affirm that oat bran is a foodstuff that helps us to lose weight and by doing this it works to protect us from many cancers.

Direct protection takes place inside us as oat bran, when consumed in sufficient quantities, forms a gel inside the digestive tract and gets mixed in with our food. It passes into and distends the stomach, then ends up in the small intestine where it takes what it can and eventually reaches the colon.

Here it not only helps give shape and consistency to the stools, but it also deposits itself on the walls of the colon. It behaves like a semi-insulating protective sheath, creating a screen between high-risk carcinogenic products and the colon's wall.

Today it is known that after the age of 40 a substantial proportion of the population develops small polyps in the intestines, tiny benign tumours that are not serious but which gastroenterologists remove as a precaution. They know that prolonged contact with high-risk or carcinogenic substances can transform these polyps into cancer.

It is estimated that it normally takes seven years for a dangerous polyp to turn into a cancer and, when assessing this risk, pollution and processed foods both have a large role to play.

So, to counteract the extreme processing our food undergoes and the ever greater amounts of suspect or downright carcinogenic products it contains, three tablespoonfuls of oat bran daily are a way of making the intestinal bolus safer and of forming a screen for the mucous membrane in the colon.

In practice, taking bran to prevent cancer only makes sense if you have good reason to suspect that the disease runs in the family or there is some likelihood of you getting it. If this is not the case and there are no other associated factors, it is unhelpful to let a fear of falling ill dictate how you live and eat, unless you love these homely cereals.

What is actually far more alarming is to note how the risk of becoming overweight can only continue to increase in the decades to come; how diabetes, obesity's closest companion, is already escalating; and how in the West the heart has become a high-risk organ, especially for those people who smoke and lead a sedentary lifestyle.

In this context, where there is a correlation between all these major health risks, oat bran really comes into its own as a foodstuff that can offer resistance against these potential pathologies. And since oat bran is not medication or some offputting potion but one of the most pleasant and helpful cereals there is, I can only campaign for it to become part of our regular eating habits.

Oat bran and constipation

Constipation is certainly a disease of our modern civilization, as is being overweight, having high cholesterol, diabetes and even cancer. It is by far the least worrying but at the same time it is the most widespread condition and women suffer from it more than men. It is a disease of civilization on two counts: with regard to actual bowel contents – the food consumed – as well as the container, the gut itself, and both play their part in slowing down bowel movement.

The food we eat today is becoming further and further removed from natural food, the food adapted to humans, to our environment and to our original physiology. For a long time our daily diet was home-grown and home-cooked. Nowadays 70 per cent of what we eat has been processed in a factory.

Industrial processing is a mixture of physical and chemical processes and, one way or another, some loss of structure or consistency is almost inevitable. This is similar to the food being pre-digested.

Tinned tuna, for example, is exactly the type of product that has lost its natural structure. Taking fresh tuna, subjecting it to industrial processing and then canning it will change its texture considerably; the firm fish flesh will go mushy. The same is true for any type of tinned food, including vegetables, which lose their texture. Tinned asparagus is tenderer than fresh asparagus; this alters its palatability and the pleasure we get from eating it, although some people prefer it this way. However, this change in texture also affects the way the food withstands being chewed, digested and absorbed.

Anything done to prepare, cook or preserve a food subjects it to processing in order to ensure that it will keep and that it can be stored to be sold at a later date. What's more, the impact of additives, prolonged cooking and salting adds up, so that the food's natural resistance gets broken down. Finally, having to market the food and ensure that it is easily consumable and attractively presented further intensifies this industrial processing. Commercially produced fruit or vegetable juice provides the most eloquent example. Orange juice is a liquid produced by squeezing the fruit, the orange's organic and plant structure is filtered and gets left behind. Yet it is precisely in this pulp that the fibre is concentrated and removing it from the fruit robs it of its structure, its consistency and its resistance.

Exactly the same may be said of most cooked meats, cheeses, tinned foods, starchy foods, pastries, confectionery, savoury and sweet biscuits. The word 'biscuit' in French means something that has been cooked twice.

When you eat processed foods they go on the same journey through your digestive system as natural food. They undergo the same mechanical treatment in the stomach and the enzymes get to work on them in the small intestine. The large colon is meant to receive unabsorbable fibre and waste saturated with water; what ends up here instead is a meagre, dehydrated bolus that does not offer enough purchase for the colon's contractions to push the contents forward. This stagnation is what we call constipation.

As for the container, the actual digestive tract, its motility and its secretions are also disrupted by our so-called post-modern civilization and its often anxiety-inducing lifestyle and environment.

How can suffering adversity slow down the digestive process in civilized human beings?

Along with the back, the digestive tract is one of the parts of the body most susceptible to stress and lack of satisfaction. Biologists know that a rat put under stress by having a painless clip attached to its tail will develop a stomach ulcer in a matter of a few weeks. So, the stomach gets psychosomatic ulcers, but the colon in particular suffers from colitis, bloating, meteorism (distension of the abdomen with air or gas) and flatulence, acting like a drum that resonates with each aggravation and frustration.

In just over a few decades there has been a spectacular increase in the incidence of spasmodic colitis. Bloating and spasms cause painful hypermotility (overactivity) in the intestines.

The intestines are circular muscles and their gentle, rhythmic contractions push the intestinal bolus forwards. However, when the contractions become irregular, the bolus gets stuck, causing tension and disrupting the digestive secretions, and this creates gas, bloating, painful cramps and rumbling noises.

Spasmodic colitis is like having a tourniquet constricting the colon at different points, slowing down and even interrupting any movement through it. The fact that antidepressants and tranquillizers can alleviate the main symptoms of painful constipation suggests that there are underlying psychological causes.

Gastroenterologists see constipation as a genuine disease of our modern civilization, an indicator of the stress generated by taking on ever more tasks and responsibilities, particularly true for women over the past 50 years. For my part, I consider that being overweight is just as much a modern disease.

And oat bran?

As a natural foodstuff, containing the best soluble fibre we know, oat bran can once again prove its role as a health-giving food.

After leaving the small intestine, where it has managed to steal away some nutrients and calories, the bran, mixed in with the remaining food bolus, enters the colon via the caecum. It travels from one end of the colon to the other, up the ascending (right) colon, crossing the tranverse colon and down the descending (left) colon until it reaches the rectal ampulla. Here the bran is expelled from the body in the stools.

All the time that it is moving through the colon, the bran fibre is, because of its solubility, soaked with water and full of calories removed from the small intestine. The colon's job is to dry out the intestinal bolus so that it can be turned into stools. However, the bran's vacuole fibre is sufficiently saturated with water for it to resist being dried out, so enough water remains to keep the stools moist.

The stools therefore remain moist and malleable because of the oat bran and its fibre. The contractions in the colon are able to gain some hold and find sufficient resistance to move the stools along.

This is how oat bran promotes bowel regularity in a completely natural way. And it works in a very different way from wheat bran, which is so well known for tackling constipation. The difference lies in the fibre. Wheat bran fibre is insoluble so it cannot absorb much water. It bulks up the stools and its fibre has a laxative effect. It is contra-indicated for all sensitive colons as it increases flatulence, bloating and painful abdominal distension.

Oat bran, on the other hand, which in solution turns into a gel, works very gently as it simply moistens the stools and maintains their volume. It works in the following cases:

- Women who are stressed and struggling to keep up with the pace of modern life, who feed themselves with overrefined, ready-to-eat foods such as white rice, white flour, white bread, freeze-dried potato granules, biscuits, breakfast cereals and filtered fruit juices – all foodstuffs that have, in effect, been pre-digested, have had their core removed and have lost much of their natural texture.

- Anyone leading a sedentary lifestyle, who does not have sufficiently taut and toned abdominal muscles to press down on their insides and move things along.
- Anyone with too much motility in the bowels; when they feel stressed and dissatisfied their bowels go into spasm and tense up.
- Where the food consumed lacks goodness because production methods require it to be simple and profitable; the food is stripped of its natural, tough structure and becomes too salty, too sugary and too fatty.
- Where the food contains too many tempting flavours designed to hook those who crave exciting taste sensations. This results in a low-level addiction to gratifying, comfort food, to the exclusion of all foods that are more natural and more in keeping with what our ancestors were programmed to eat.

Eating such food testifies to a need for taste sensations that in itself reveals an alarming need to compensate for dissatisfaction and a conflict between our basic human nature and an environment in turmoil. This gap between our real needs and the lives we lead in practice is one of the greatest problems confronting modern humanity.

The world is very busy tending to our ailing environment and ecology. Institutions, political parties, governments, philosophers and even religious leaders try to outdo each other with ideas about how to protect the environment and ensure sustainable production. This is all excellent! But who is talking about human ecology?

Who is concerned about our capacity to adapt, as we exhaust ourselves acclimatizing to a toxic, artificial and unnatural way of life? We have enjoyed using the wheel, the pitchfork and pottery. We were dazzled by the steam engine, filled with enthusiasm for electricity. Then we became dependent on needs invented wholly through advances in technology, such as cars, trains and the cinema. Then the first double-edged innovations appeared, those that brought as much benefit as harm, such as mass production, television and even the telephone, which makes communication easier but also leads to increased physical separation.

And finally, at an even faster rate, 'false' needs appeared on the scene, innovations to entertain us that do more harm than good, temptations that seduce us but which only generate surface satisfaction and do not get to the simple heart of what brings us real contentment.

You can never do away with an invention. I am only campaigning and speaking out for what I call 'human ecology' to appear alongside environmental ecology. Its aim would be simply to promote the individual's happiness and well-being. This apparently utopian objective is simple: all we need to do is identify genuine human needs, those that we can easily and naturally satisfy. And then start by making sure that these are satisfied before we become addicted to any others that offer us only surface satisfaction, stimulating by virtue of their novelty but transient, so they fade away again very quickly and without even satisfying our original need.

Oat bran offers us a solution that is an integral part of this new human ecology.

A food with flavour, a reassuring food, a food that protects us from the main health dangers hanging over our lives, a food that can be easily cooked in so many different ways, a food that tackles weight problems head-on, a health-giving food – in its own way oat bran offers us satisfaction and helps us feel better in ourselves; it gives us well-being and, let's dare say the word, happiness.

Part III:

Oat bran recipes

50 ways to enjoy oat bran

Given oat bran's many impressive qualities and benefits, some people may well be thinking to themselves that to take such a panacea you will need to hold your nose as you do with cod liver oil!

This is not the case at all. Not only is oat bran a slimming and quasi-medicinal food but it is also a high-quality foodstuff with taste, flavour and consistency, and it lends itself to being used in a whole variety of dishes, each as delicious as the next.

First of all let us take a look at the actual product and how you purchase it.

Bran is the name given to the fibrous outer casing of a cereal. Just as wheat bran is the outer husk for the wheat grain, oat bran is the fibrous casing that protects the oat grain inside. All sorts of insects and parasites are very keen to devour cereals. To ensure high productivity, cereal crops are sprayed with pesticides which pollute the bran more than the grain. So like any other cereal, fruit or vegetable, oat bran is of better quality if it is grown organically using as few pesticides as possible. However, given how scarce it is nowadays, there is not enough organic oat bran available to meet demand so we will have to wait until economic pressure from consumers encourages new producers to come up with the goods.

As you look around to buy your oat bran you will notice that it comes in various forms, weights and different brands. One fact you should know is that you can get oat bran with or without the germ.

What is the germ? It is the little energy store that comes with the grain. It is the equivalent of the egg yolk, which allows the developing chick to get what it needs to keep alive. The wheat or oat grain germ plays the same role as the egg yolk, providing the grain with the stored energy it requires to survive until maturity. It will come as no surprise to you that this store, concentrated as it is into a tiny space, is high in fat.

If you are being strict about losing or controlling your weight and you have to take several tablespoonfuls each day, then you need to avoid the germ as it will bump up your calories. If you are only taking a single table-spoonful a day, or if you are taking oat bran for a reason other than being overweight, then there is no need for you to avoid the oat germ as it is made up of excellent fatty acids that are very good for your health. What is more, the germ further enhances the bran's flavour and palatability.

Some people cannot tell the difference between the two oat brans. Some prefer it without the germ but if you can taste a palpable difference in flavour then do not think twice about eating it with the germ. I cannot stress this enough – for anyone faced with controlling their weight and what they eat, pleasure is their chief ally.

Oat bran comes in different sized packs, ranging from 250g to 10kg. The ideal size is a 250g pack for individual use. One tablespoonful of oat bran weighs 10–15g. If you use three tablespoonfuls per day, that comes to about 40g a day on average so you would get through one pack a week. This allows you to keep the bran dry, thus ensuring that it not only tastes good and can add flavour, but is able to soak up water and nutrients which is its main property.

After using your oat bran seal the pack carefully, the simplest way being the traditional clothes peg. Never put oat bran in the fridge and certainly not in the freezer – you will be condemning it to a cold death!

Oat bran tastes naturally chewy. It has this consistency because it is soluble and, like pectin, is able to turn into a gel. It is not recommended that you eat oat bran dry, by the spoonful, as it will immediately become filled with saliva and stick to your mouth until it gets saturated and soaked with liquid. However, I do have some patients who enjoy eating it like this. When used with liquid – water, milk or dairy products – it soaks it up and is chewiest in milk.

Use a blender or food processor as little as possible with oat bran. You will rob it of its plant texture and many of its best properties, its density and its resistance when eaten. However, there are some recipes where the bran needs blending to become finer and chewier and more pleasurable to eat.

Oat bran has a sweetish taste; the American and Scandinavian brans taste almost sweet. This flavour comes from the beta-glucans in the bran: during cooking they become concentrated, increasing the beta-glucan content and, on the surface of a galette cooked over a hot plate, a slightly caramelized film is formed. Some cooks make this film thicker by adding pumpkin powder. The natural sweetness comes through best when the mixture used is very thin, such as crêpes made with milk which can often be enjoyed just as they are without any additional sugar or sweetener.

If you are not watching your weight, you can sweeten the bran in cakes with table sugar. If you are overweight you can use aspartame to sweeten the mixtures you prepare. However, do be aware that if you then cook your mixture at a high temperature or for a long time, aspartame's sweetness will fade. In this case it is better not to use sweetener in your galette and crêpe mixtures, but once they are cooked sprinkle your sweetener over them.

Spices may also be added. The most popular ones are cinnamon, vanilla and orange flower. Always go for the actual spices rather than their flavourings. Nonetheless, powdered or syrup flavourings are very practical; it is always best to opt for natural flavourings rather than the synthetic ones. For example, do not spoil your oat bran with industrially manufactured vanillin. You should also try ginger as it tastes wonderful in galettes.

For savoury mixtures, ideally you would add some dried herbes de Provence. Once cooked, they turn out to be a great flavour enhancer, providing texture and a lovely 'crunchiness', and they will add a little sophistication to your galettes.

Finally, sprinkling some well toasted sesame seeds into your mixture will taste delicious too!

Recipe notes

- Eggs are medium and preferably free-range. Some recipes are made with raw or lightly cooked eggs: pregnant or breast-feeding women, invalids, the elderly and very young children should avoid these dishes.
- Both metric and imperial measurements have been given – do not use a mixture of both but stick to one set.
- Spoon measures are level unless otherwise stated. 1 tablespoon = 15ml, 1 teaspoon = 5ml.
- Some recipes contain nut flavourings – those with known allergic reactions to nuts and nut derivatives, pregnant and breast-feeding women and very young children should avoid these dishes.

MY FLAGSHIP RECIPES:
SWEET AND SAVOURY GALETTES

As I wrote at the beginning of this book, the idea of using oat bran was born out of the love that connects me to my daughter Maya.

For her and thanks to her, I devised the galette which provided my method with what it was missing – an ultra slow, tasty, filling and slimming carbohydrate, one that is easy to cook with and quasi-medicinal as it protects our health in the four areas where Westerners are at risk today.

As it all started with the galette – with sweet or rather sweetened galettes for some and savoury galettes for others – I have decided to give the galette centre stage by devoting a separate section to it before adding a string of other recipes.

If you are overweight and dieting, you can imagine just how useful it is to have this carbohydrate to liven up your diet, curb your appetite and allow your culinary imagination a free rein.

If you are diabetic, you can eat a slow carbohydrate that will be absorbed only gradually, that tastes like bread and has the texture of a pancake or blini without you having to fret over the nagging question of portion control.

If you are constipated, your bowel movements will very gently become more comfortable and fluid as your circular bowel muscles have something to push on to get things moving.

If you have high cholesterol, take a note of the date and get yourself tested two months after you start eating oat bran – the results will surprise you.

And if you suffer from none of these complaints, just enjoy eating the bran and tell yourself that you stand a very good chance of escaping them for a long time to come.

As for you, dear readers, if your imagination leads you to discover a new recipe or a new use for oat bran, please be kind enough to let me know and I promise to name it after you.

SWEET GALETTE

Sweet galettes are delicious flavoured with vanilla, cinnamon or orange flower (water).

Preparation time: 1 minute
Cooking time: 2–3 minutes
1 serving

1½ tablespoons oat bran
1½ tablespoons fat-free fromage frais
1 egg white or 1 whole egg depending on your
    medical instructions
Artificial sweetener, e.g. aspartame, or 1 teaspoon
    Hermesetas

Combine all the basic ingredients until the mixture is smooth, and add the sweetener. Pour into a frying pan, warmed over a medium heat, and cook for about 1–2 minutes. Using a spatula, turn the galette over and cook for the same time on the other side.

TIP Sweet galettes can be eaten as pancakes. If you add a little milk to make the mixture runnier, you can produce thinner crêpes. You can make chocolate brownies, too, with fat-reduced cocoa powder or, if you are not watching your weight, Van Houten-type cocoa powder. You can make biscuits from a galette, using a knife, biscuit cutter or a sharp-edged glass to cut out the shapes. Place the biscuits on a baking sheet and bake at 220°C/425°F/Gas 7 for 5 minutes on each side.

SAVOURY GALETTE

Savoury galettes can be eaten like bread and used to make up a sandwich. Or you can eat them as a blini topped with a slice of smoked salmon, or lean cooked ham, chicken or turkey.

Preparation time: 1 minute
Cooking time: 2–3 minutes
1 serving

1½ tablespoons oat bran
1½ tablespoons fat-free fromage frais
1 egg white or 1 whole egg depending on your
    medical instructions
Herbes de Provence
Salt and black pepper

Combine all the basic ingredients until the mixture is smooth. Add herbs and seasoning to taste. Pour into a frying pan, warmed over a medium heat, and cook for about 1–2 minutes. Using a spatula, turn the galette over and cook for the same time on the other side.

TIP You can also use a savoury galette as a pizza base. There is a wide range of toppings to choose from; for example, tuna (in brine or spring water) is particularly nice with fresh or puréed tomato, a few capers and a little low-fat cream cheese spread over the top to finish off.

SAVOURY RECIPES

COURGETTE AND FETA APPETIZERS
(BOUCHÉES DE COURGETTE ET DE FETA)

These appetizers also make a perfect accompaniment for roast chicken or émincé of chicken.

Preparation time: 10 minutes
Cooking time: 30 minutes
Makes 20 appetizers

1 courgette
1 onion, thinly sliced
½ bunch of basil, finely chopped
100g (3½oz) feta cheese (9% fat), crumbled
3 tablespoons oat bran
2 eggs
Salt and black pepper

Preheat the oven to 220°C/425°F/Gas 7.

Grate the courgette without peeling it. In a large bowl, combine the courgette with the remaining ingredients. Once the mixture is well blended, spoon out in small balls and place on a baking sheet covered with greaseproof paper. Bake in the preheated oven for 15 minutes then turn the appetizers over and bake for a further 15 minutes.

CRAB AND PRAWN LOAF
(CAKE AU CRABE ET AUX CREVETTES)

Preparation time: 10 minutes
Cooking time: 35 minutes
4 servings

4 eggs
8 tablespoons oat bran
3 tablespoons wheat bran
1 × 8g sachet baking powder
6 tablespoons skimmed milk powder
1 × 170g can crab meat, flaked
200g (7oz) prawns
2 teaspoons mustard
Salt and black pepper

Preheat the oven to 200°C/400°F/Gas 6 for 15 minutes then reduce to 180°C/350°F/Gas 4.

In a bowl, mix together 2 whole eggs with 2 egg yolks, retaining the whites. Add all the remaining ingredients. Whisk the 2 egg whites until stiff and fold them into the mixture. Tip the mixture into a tin and bake in the preheated oven for 35 minutes.

MUSHROOM AND HAM LOAF
(CAKE FORESTIER)

Preparation time: 20 minutes
Cooking time: 35 minutes
4 servings

175g (6oz) mixed mushrooms
150g (5½oz) smoked ham, cut into thin strips
4 eggs
4 tablespoons fat-free fromage frais
8 tablespoons oat bran
3 tablespoons wheat bran
6 tablespoons skimmed milk powder
A few shallots, finely chopped
Black pepper – but no salt!
1 × 8g sachet baking powder

Preheat the oven to 200°C/400°F/Gas 6 for 15 minutes then reduce to 180°C/350°F/Gas 4.

Gently fry the mushrooms and smoked ham in a frying pan to remove all the water. Leave to cool.

In the meantime, mix together in a bowl 2 whole eggs and 2 yolks, retaining the whites. Add the fromage frais, oat and wheat brans, skimmed milk powder and seasonings. Whisk the 2 egg whites until stiff and fold them into the mixture. Stir in the cooled ham and mushrooms then add the baking powder. Mix together very thoroughly, tip into a tin and bake in the preheated oven for 35 minutes.

CHICKEN TURNOVER
(CHAUSSON AU POULET)

Preparation time: 2–3 minutes
Cooking time: 2–3 minutes
1 serving

1 savoury Dukan galette (see p.108)
Extra-light cream cheese (4–6% fat)
Black pepper
1 slice cooked chicken

Make a savoury galette following the recipe on p.108 then spread it with the cream cheese, grind over some black pepper and add a slice of cooked chicken. Fold the galette to make a turnover and cook it again, briefly, on both sides.

SMOKED SALMON AND PRAWN TURNOVER (CHAUSSON AUX CREVETTES ET AU SAUMON)

Preparation time: 5 minutes
Cooking time: 2–3 minutes
1 serving

2 egg whites
2 tablespoons oat bran
1 tablespoon wheat bran
Fromage frais
1 small bowl prawns, cooked
1 tablespoon extra-light cream cheese (4–6% fat)
3 slices smoked salmon
A few shallots, chopped (optional)
Parsley, to serve (optional)

Whisk the egg whites until stiff. Fold in the oat and wheat brans, a tiny bit of fromage frais and the prawns. Cook the galette. Once you have cooked both sides, spread the galette with the tablespoonful of extra-light cream cheese, add the smoked salmon slices and fold to make a turnover. You can also add some chopped shallots and fresh parsley.

HAM, EGG AND CHEESE CRÊPE (CRÊPE COMPLÈTE)

Preparation time: 15 minutes
Cooking time: 6–7 minutes
1 serving

½ tablespoon cornflour
200ml (7fl oz) skimmed milk
2 slices turkey ham
30g (1oz) grated cheese (6% fat)
2 eggs
2 tablespoons oat bran
1 tablespoon wheat bran
Salt and black pepper

First make a thick Dukan béchamel sauce by combining the cornflour with half the cold skimmed milk. Warm the mixture in a pan for a few minutes over a gentle heat, stirring continually as it thickens, then season with salt and black pepper.

Place the two slices of turkey ham in a microwavable dish, cover with the grated cheese and break one of the eggs on top. Place a lid over the dish and microwave until the egg white is cooked (about 2 minutes).

In a bowl combine the oat bran, wheat bran, 5 tablespoons of skimmed milk and the remaining egg. Very lightly oil a non-stick frying pan, spread the mixture out so that the crêpe is thin and cook on both sides. Spread the béchamel sauce over the crêpe, smoothing it over with the back of a spoon. Then, using a large spatula, place the turkey ham and cooked egg on top. Fold over the edges of the crêpe and finish off with some freshly ground black pepper.

HAM AND MUSHROOM PANCAKES (FICELLES PICARDES)

Preparation time: 20 minutes
Cooking time: 10 minutes
2 servings

2 savoury Dukan galettes (see p.108)
Handful of cooked button mushrooms
Dukan béchamel sauce (see above)
1 slice cooked ham, cut in half
Extra-light cream cheese (optional)
5% fat crème fraîche or fat-free fromage frais

Make the galettes following the recipe on p.108 but replace the fromage frais with 1½ tablespoons milk. Add a few cooked mushrooms to the béchamel sauce. Place one half of the sliced ham on top of each galette along with a large spoonful of the mushroom sauce and, if you like, a little extra-light cream cheese. Roll up the crêpes and place them in an oven dish. Cover with a little crème fraîche or fromage frais and bake in the oven for 10 minutes.

FRESH SALMON AND FROMAGE FRAIS GALETTE (GALETTE AU FROMAGE FRAIS ET AU SAUMON)

Preparation time: 30 minutes
Cooking time: 15 minutes
1 serving

100g (3½oz) virtually fat-free quark
200g (7oz) filleted fresh salmon
1 tablespoon lemon juice
2 teaspoons mixed herbs of your choice, plus extra
2 tablespoons oat bran
1 tablespoon wheat bran
1 egg
2 tablespoons fat-free fromage frais
1 teaspoon paprika
Spices of your choice (e.g. cumin, paprika, celery
    powder)
Salt and black pepper

While you prepare the dish, leave the quark to drain on some kitchen paper.

Season the salmon with the lemon juice, 1 teaspoon mixed herbs, salt and black pepper, then steam it for 10 minutes.

Meanwhile, make a galette: mix together the oat bran, wheat bran, egg, fromage frais, paprika, a pinch of salt and 1 teaspoon mixed herbs. Season the drained quark with salt and black pepper, herbs and spices of your choice. Cook the galette in a frying pan over a medium heat for 1–2 minutes on each side, then spread over the quark and top with the steamed salmon fillet.

TUNA GALETTE
(GALETTE AU THON)

Preparation time: 10 minutes
Cooking time: 20 minutes
1 serving

Ingredients for 1 savoury Dukan galette (see p.108)
½ × 185g can tuna, crushed with a fork
1 egg
Handful of spring onions, chopped

Preheat the oven to 180°C/350°F/Gas 4.

Prepare the savoury galette following the recipe on p.108 and stir the tuna into the mixture. Add the egg and spring onions and bake in the preheated oven in a small dish for 20 minutes. Cooking times may vary depending on the oven.

BRESAOLA GALETTE
(GALETTE À LA VIANDE DES GRISONS)

Preparation time: 5 minutes
Cooking time: 4–5 minutes
1 serving

1 savoury Dukan galette (see p.108)
5–6 slices bresaola
1 tablespoon extra-light cream cheese (5% fat)

Make the galette base following the recipe on p.108. Once it is cooked arrange the bresaola slices and cream cheese on top and place under a preheated grill until it turns golden brown.

GALETTE WITH MARINATED HERRINGS AND MIXED SALAD (GALETTE DE HARENGS MARINÉS ET SALADE MÉLANGÉE)

Preparation time: 5 minutes
Cooking time: 2–3 minutes
1 serving

1 savoury Dukan galette (see p.108)
1 carrot, thinly sliced
½ onion, thinly sliced
100g (3½oz) mild smoked herring
5 peppercorn mix
150g (5½oz) mixed salad

First make a savoury galette following the recipe on p.108. Mix together the sliced carrot and onion with the smoked herring. Spread this mixture generously over the galette and grind some of the peppercorn mix over the top. Serve with the mixed salad.

CARBONARA-STYLE OAT GNOCCHI (GNOCCHIS D'AVOINE FAÇON CARBONARA)

Preparation time: 35 minutes
Cooking time: 5 minutes
1 serving

1 tablespoon wheat bran
3 tablespoons oat bran
1½ tablespoons fat-free fromage frais
1 teaspoon cornflour
100ml (3½fl oz) skimmed milk
1 low-salt stock cube
1 slice lean smoked ham
1 egg yolk
Salt and black pepper

Use a blender to blend the wheat bran and the oat bran until they are as fine as possible. Add a pinch of salt and the fat-free fromage frais. Knead the mixture for a couple of minutes then shape it into a ball. Leave the dough to rest for 5 minutes.

Prepare a béchamel sauce by mixing the cornflour into the cold skimmed milk, and sprinkle in a third of the stock cube. Warm for a few minutes over a gentle heat, stirring continuously while the sauce thickens, then season with black pepper. Bring a large pan of water to the boil with the rest of the stock cube sprinkled in.

Meanwhile, cut the dough ball into quarters then take one piece and roll it between your hands to form a long thin sausage. Lay it flat on a plate and cut into 1.5cm (5/8in) long sections to make your gnocchi. Repeat with the remaining dough quarters. Chop the ham into small cubes and gently fry in a non-stick pan. Add the béchamel sauce. Tip the gnocchi into the boiling water and, once they rise to the surface, cook for 1 minute. Remove them from the pan and place on some kitchen paper to drain off.

To serve, stir the gnocchi into the béchamel sauce and stir in the egg yolk.

THE DUKAN BURGER

Preparation time: 10 minutes
Cooking time: 5 minutes
1 serving

1 savoury Dukan galette (see p.108)
1 teaspoon mustard
1 beef burger (5% fat), cooked
½ onion, sliced
1 lettuce leaf
1 fried egg
Salt and black pepper

First make a savoury galette following the recipe on p.108. Spread some mustard over it, add the burger, onion slices, lettuce and fried egg, and season with salt and black pepper to taste.

THE DUKAN HOT-DOG

Preparation time: 5 minutes
Cooking time: 1–2 minutes
1 serving

1 savoury Dukan galette (see p.108)
2 turkey sausages
A little French mustard

Prepare a savoury galette following the recipe on p.108. Place the turkey sausages on top, spread with a little French mustard then roll up into a hot-dog and eat!

DUKAN BREAD
(PAIN DUKAN)

Preparation time: 5 minutes
Cooking time: 10 minutes
1 serving

1 egg
15g (½oz) fat-free fromage frais
15g (½oz) virtually fat-free quark
1 level tablespoon cornflour
1 teaspoon baking powder
Dried herbs of your choice – but no salt!

Preheat the oven to 200°C/400°F/Gas 6, or use the microwave.

Combine all the ingredients and pour them into a 15cm (6in) x 20cm (8in) rectangular dish. The mixture should be at least 5mm (¼in) thick. Cover with clingfilm and place in the microwave on the maximum setting for 5 minutes. Alternatively bake in the preheated oven for at least 10 minutes (without any clingfilm).

Once the bread is cooked, remove the clingfilm immediately if using the microwave, and turn it out of the dish so that it does not collapse.

DUKAN PAN BAGNAT

Preparation time: 5 minutes
1 serving

For the galette
1 savoury Dukan galette (see p.108)
1 × ?g can tuna (in brine or spring water)
A few capers
1 lettuce leaf
1–2 slices tomato

For the Dukan mayonnaise
1 egg yolk
Spices
Tabasco
1–2 tablespoons fat-free fromage frais
Vinegar

First prepare a savoury galette following the recipe on p.108.

Make the mayonnaise by whisking the egg yolk with the spices. Add 2 drops of Tabasco and then the fromage frais as if it were oil, whisking all the time. Finish off with a drizzle of vinegar.

Combine the tuna, capers, lettuce and tomato slices, and spread over the cooked galette.

MOZZARELLA PANINI
(PANINI À LA MOZZARELLA)

Preparation time: 5 minutes
Cooking time: 5–6 minutes
1 serving

2 tablespoons oat bran
1 tablespoon wheat bran
3 tablespoons skimmed milk powder
2 eggs
10 drops butter flavouring (www.mydukandietshop.
 co.uk)
1 teaspoon baking powder
1 low-fat mozzarella ball (9% fat), sliced
½ tomato, thinly sliced
4 slices bresaola
Salt and black pepper

First make the base. In a bowl, mix together the oat
bran, wheat bran, skimmed milk powder, eggs, butter
flavouring and baking powder. Lightly oil a non-stick
frying pan. Cook the base for 30 seconds, making sure
it is a nice, large rectangular shape. Then, using a spatula, turn the base over and turn off the heat. Cut the
base in half lengthways.

Heat the mozzarella slices under the grill for a few
minutes to get rid of any excess water. Arrange the
tomato over one half of the base. Add the bresaola

slices and cover with the melted mozzarella. Season with salt and black pepper. Place the other half of the base on top, then grill the panini in a sandwich toaster until nice and crispy on the outside.

CHICKEN AND RED PEPPER PIZZA
(PIZZA AU POULET ET AU POIVRON ROUGE)

Preparation time: 20 minutes
Cooking time: 10 minutes
2 servings

4 heaped tablespoons oat bran
2 heaped tablespoons wheat bran
3 tablespoons skimmed milk powder
4 egg whites (retain 1 yolk)
2 eggs
½ teaspoon walnut flavouring (www.
    mydukandietshop.co.uk)
1 red pepper, thinly sliced
1 teaspoon olive oil
150g (5½oz) virtually fat-free quark
50ml (2fl oz) crème fraîche (3% fat)
4 tablespoons chopped tomatoes
1 large cooked chicken breast, chopped
A little grated low-fat Gruyère
Salt and black pepper

First make the pizza base. In a bowl, mix together the oat bran, wheat bran, skimmed milk powder, the 4 egg whites, the 2 whole eggs and the walnut flavouring. Season with salt and black pepper. Lightly oil a large non-stick frying pan, pour in the mixture and cook for 40 seconds on each side.

Preheat the oven to 180°C/350°F/Gas 4.

Gently fry the sliced red pepper in a non-stick frying pan with the olive oil and 2 tablespoons of water. Stir occasionally until the liquid evaporates.

In a bowl, combine the virtually fat-free quark, crème fraîche, chopped tomatoes and egg yolk. Check the seasoning but do not use too much.

Place the pizza base on a baking sheet covered with aluminium foil and spread the quark mixture over it. Scatter the chopped cooked chicken, sliced pepper and Gruyère on top. Season with salt and black pepper and bake in the preheated oven for 10 minutes.

SALMON AND CHEESE PIZZA
(PIZZA AU SAUMON ET AU FROMAGE)

Preparation time: 20 minutes
Cooking time: 10 minutes
1 serving

3 tablespoons oat bran
3 tablespoons skimmed milk powder
1 egg
1 egg white
70g (2½oz) virtually fat-free quark
100g (3½oz) smoked salmon
1 tablespoon crème fraîche (3% fat)
1 Bridelight melting cheese (2% fat), diced
Salt and black pepper

Preheat the oven to 180°C/350°F/Gas 4.

First make the pizza base. In a bowl, mix together the oat bran, skimmed milk powder, whole egg, egg white and some black pepper, Using some kitchen paper, very lightly oil a non-stick frying pan. Cook the base for 30 seconds on each side, turning it over with a spatula (the mixture should still look runny). Place the pizza base on a baking sheet covered with aluminium foil and spread it generously with the quark. Place the smoked salmon on top with the crème fraîche, and scatter over the cheese. Bake in the preheated oven for 10 minutes, keeping a careful eye on the pizza. When it's ready, season to taste and serve hot.

SMOKED SALMON AND LEEK PIZZA (PIZZA AU SAUMON ET AUX POIREAUX)

Preparation time: 10 minutes
Cooking time: 10 minutes
2 servings

4 heaped tablespoons oat bran
2 heaped tablespoons wheat bran
3 tablespoons skimmed milk powder
2 eggs
4 egg whites
½ teaspoon walnut flavouring (www.
mydukandietshop.co.uk)
150g (5½oz) virtually fat-free quark
100ml (3½fl oz) crème fraîche (3% fat), plus extra
4 leeks (white part only), thinly sliced
3 slices smoked salmon
2 Emmental cheeses, diced
Salt and black pepper

Preheat the oven to 180°C/350°F/Gas 4.

First make the pizza base. Mix together in a bowl the oat bran, wheat bran, skimmed milk powder, eggs, egg whites and walnut flavouring. Season with salt and black pepper. Very lightly oil a large non-stick frying pan. Pour in the pizza mixture and cook for 40 seconds on each side, turning it over with a spatula (the mixture should still look runny).

In another bowl mix together the quark and crème fraîche, and season with a little salt and black pepper. Spread this mixture over the pizza base and place on a baking sheet covered with aluminium foil. Next arrange the leek whites on top, together with the smoked salmon and cheese. Finish off by dotting the pizza with some extra crème fraîche and season. Bake in the preheated oven for 10 minutes.

TUNA PIZZA
(PIZZA AU THON)

Preparation time: 20 minutes
Cooking time: 10 minutes
1 serving

1 savoury Dukan galette (see p.108)
1 large onion, chopped
1 × 400g can chopped tomatoes, drained
1 teaspoon thyme, oregano and basil
2 pinches of Cayenne pepper
175g (6oz) canned tuna (in brine or spring water),
    drained
2 tablespoons capers
60g (2¼oz) extra-light cream cheese
Salt

Use a savoury galette as your pizza base. Gently fry the onion in a frying pan. Add the tomatoes, herbs and Cayenne pepper, then season with a little salt. Leave the sauce to simmer and thicken, over a gentle heat, for 10 minutes. Flake the tuna into a bowl and put to one side. Spread the tomato sauce over the galette, scatter over the tuna and capers and dot with the extra-light cream cheese. Eat straightaway.

OCEAN PIZZA
(PIZZA OCÉANE)

Preparation time: 5 minutes
Cooking time: 10 minutes
1 serving

For the pizza
1 tablespoon wheat bran
2 tablespoons oat bran
⅔ tablespoon fat-free fromage frais
3 tablespoons skimmed milk powder
1 egg (or 1 egg white)
Salt and black pepper

For the topping
70g (2½oz) virtually fat-free quark
100g (3½oz) trout, cooked
3–4 scallops, cooked
100g (3½oz) small prawns, cooked
Fresh dill
1 teaspoon mustard
1 tablespoon fat-free fromage frais
Juice of 1 lemon
Salt and black pepper

Preheat the oven to 200°C/400°F/Gas 6.

First make the pizza base by mixing together all the ingredients in a bowl. Roll out on some greaseproof paper into a pizza shape, the size of a standard round plate, and bake on a tray in the middle of the preheated oven for a few minutes, until the pizza turns golden brown. Once it is ready, spread over the quark, and arrange the trout, scallops, prawns and dill on top. Stir the mustard into the fromage frais, then dot this mixture over the pizza and drizzle over a little lemon juice. Season to taste. Warm the pizza under a preheated grill for a few minutes.

ORIENTAL PIZZA
(PIZZA ORIENTALE)

Preparation time: 20 minutes
Cooking time: 10 minutes
2 servings

4 heaped tablespoons oat bran
2 heaped tablespoons wheat bran
3 tablespoons skimmed milk powder
4 eggs
4 egg whites
½ teaspoon walnut flavouring (www.
   mydukandietshop.co.uk)
200g minced steak (5% fat)
1 large onion, finely chopped
½ × 40g can tomato purée
Ground cumin
150g (5½oz) virtually fat-free quark
50ml (2fl oz) crème fraîche (3% fat)
A little grated low-fat Gruyère
Salt and black pepper

Start off by making the pizza base. In a bowl, mix together the oat bran, wheat bran, skimmed milk powder, 3 of the eggs, the 4 egg whites and the walnut flavouring. Season with salt and black pepper.

Very lightly oil a large non-stick frying pan, pour in the mixture and cook for 40 seconds on each side.

Preheat the oven to 180°C/350°F/Gas 4.

Combine the minced beef with the remaining egg, the onion and 4 tablespoons of the tomato purée. Add salt and black pepper and a pinch of ground cumin. Gently fry in a non-stick frying pan until lightly browned then put to one side.

In a bowl, combine the quark and crème fraîche. Add some salt and black pepper but take care not to overseason. Finish off with a little ground cumin.

Place the pizza base on a baking sheet that has been covered with aluminium foil and spread the quark mixture over it. Add the rest of the tomato purée to the minced beef mixture and spread this over the pizza. Scatter a little grated low-fat Gruyère over the top. Season with salt and black pepper and bake in the preheated oven for 10 minutes.

HERBY CHICKEN ROLLS
(ROULÉS DE POULET AUX HERBES)

Preparation time: 5 minutes
Cooking time: 10 minutes
1 serving

1 savoury Dukan galette (see p.108)
1 thin chicken breast
Handful of thinly sliced button mushrooms
½ garlic clove, crushed
50g (1¾oz) virtually fat-free quark
1 tablespoon chives, chopped
1 tablespoon flat parsley, chopped
Salt and black pepper

Make a savoury galette following the recipe on p.108, cut it in half and put to one side. Using a rolling pin, flatten out the chicken breast and slice it in two lengthways. Very lightly oil a non-stick frying pan and cook both pieces of chicken for 5 minutes on both sides until they are golden brown.

To prepare the stuffing, fry the mushrooms in a frying pan together with the crushed garlic. Leave to cool down, then add the quark, chives and parsley. Season with salt and black pepper and mix all the ingredients together thoroughly. Place a piece of chicken breast on each half of the galette, then add a large spoonful of the stuffing, roll up and hold together with a cocktail stick.

OAT BRAN SPAGHETTI WITH BOLOGNAISE SAUCE (SPAGHETTIS DE SON À LA BOLOGNAISE)

Preparation time: 20 minutes
Cooking time: 10 minutes
2 servings

For the spaghetti
2 tablespoons oat bran
1 tablespoon wheat bran
1 egg
3 tablespoons skimmed milk powder
2 teaspoons fat-free fromage frais
Butter flavouring (www.mydukandietshop.co.uk)
Salt, to taste
Approx. 20g (1oz) Protifar protein powder

For the sauce
200g minced steak (5% fat)
½ onion, thinly sliced
1 small carrot, finely diced (optional)
Olive flavouring (www.mydukandietshop.co.uk)
40g (1½oz) lardons or diced bacon
150g (5½oz) tomato purée
Plenty of herbs (e.g. herbes de Provence or parsley)
1 garlic clove, crushed
Salt and black pepper
A little grated low-fat Gruyère, to serve (optional)

In a large bowl, mix all the spaghetti ingredients together, adding the protein powder at the last moment, until the dough becomes 'non-sticky'. Sprinkle a little protein powder on to a wooden chopping board, then roll out the dough (if it sticks to the rolling pin use your fingers). Take a large, non-serrated knife and cut into long strips by placing the blade on to the dough, pressing down then removing it. Keep going in one direction, so the dough does not get broken up, until it is all cut into spaghetti-like strips.

Place the spaghetti strips in a large pan and cover with hot, salted water. Turn on the heat and wait for the water to start bubbling. In the meantime, place some kitchen paper on a plate. When the spaghetti has cooked for a few minutes (it will change colour and froth will appear) gently remove using a slotted spoon and transfer on to the kitchen paper. Keep to one side.

Gently fry the mince in a frying pan, ensuring it is all broken up. Once cooked through, transfer the mince to a bowl and set aside; then add the onion and carrot (if using) to the pan along with the olive flavouring. Whenever necessary, add a little water to stop the vegetables from burning. Once the onion starts to turn translucent, add the lardons or bacon and gently fry everything. Return the mince to the pan and stir in the tomato purée. Add herbs, garlic and seasoning to taste. Cover and leave to simmer over a gentle heat for a few minutes so that all the flavours can mingle.

The Oat Bran Miracle

When ready to serve, place the spaghetti on warmed plates, pour over the bolognaise sauce and sprinkle some grated Gruyère on top if wished.

SMOKED SALMON AND COTTAGE CHEESE SLICE WITH SALAD (TARTINE DE SAUMON FUMÉ SUR LIT DE FROMAGE ET SA SALADE)

Preparation time: 10 minutes
Cooking time: 2–3 minutes
1 serving

75g cottage cheese
2 tablespoons oat bran
2 tablespoons wheat bran
1 egg
1 tablespoon fat-free fromage frais
Herbs of your choice (e.g. parsley, basil, thyme)
Spices of your choice (e.g. paprika, cumin, celery
    powder)
100g (3½oz) smoked salmon
150g (5½oz) Webbs lettuce
1 tomato, sliced
Salt and black pepper

Firstly, drain the cottage cheese for several hours until it is really thick. Then make a savoury galette by mixing together the oat and wheat brans, egg, fromage frais and seasoning, and cooking as described on p.108.

Season the cheese with some salt, black pepper, herbs and spices. Generously spread this mixture over the galette and cover with the smoked salmon. Finish off with some freshly grated black pepper and serve with a salad composed of Webbs lettuce and sliced tomato.

SEAFOOD TERRINE
(TERRINE AUX FRUITS DE MER)

Preparation time: 15 minutes
Cooking time: 30 minutes
2 servings

2 tablespoons wheat bran
4 tablespoons oat bran
3 tablespoons fat-free fromage frais
3 eggs
Generous handful of mixed seafood, fresh or frozen
Salt, black pepper and herbs, to season

Preheat the oven to 180°C/350°F/Gas 4.

Blend all the ingredients until you have a smooth mixture, then pour into a tin lined with baking paper. Bake in the preheated oven for about 30 minutes.

CREAM OF MUSHROOM SOUP WITH OAT BRAN (VELOUTÉ DE CÈPES AU SON D'AVOINE)

Preparation time: 10 minutes
Cooking time: 20 minutes
2 servings

1 small garlic clove
250g (9oz) ceps or porcini mushrooms
4 tablespoons chives, chopped
500ml (18fl oz) skimmed milk
4 tablespoons oat bran
1 egg yolk, beaten (optional)
Salt and black pepper

Roughly crush the garlic clove using the blade of a knife. Clean the mushrooms and gently fry for 10 minutes in a lightly oiled frying pan along with the garlic and chives. Blend the mushrooms and add this mixture to a pan containing the skimmed milk and oat bran. Stir continuously over a medium heat for 10 minutes. A minute before the soup is ready, add the egg yolk if it needs thickening. Season to taste with salt and black pepper, and serve.

SWEET RECIPES

CHOCOLATE CHIP BISCUITS
(BISCUITS AUX PÉPITES DE CHOCOLAT)

Preparation time: 45 minutes
Cooking time: 20 minutes
Makes approx. 15 biscuits

2 tablespoons fat-reduced cocoa powder (e.g. Van Houten)
1 egg yolk
3 tablespoons powdered sweetener
1 tablespoon wheat bran
2 tablespoons oat bran
15g (½oz) virtually fat-free quark
15g (½oz) fat-free fromage frais
1 tablespoon cornflour
1 egg
1 teaspoon baking powder
1 teaspoon vanilla extract

Make a chocolate mix by stirring the cocoa powder into the egg yolk along with 1 tablespoon of the powdered sweetener. Wrap the mixture in some cling-film and flatten it so that you end up with a fairly thick rectangular bar. Place in the freezer until it hardens.

Preheat the oven to 160°C/325°F/Gas 3.

In a bowl, combine the wheat bran with the oat bran. Cut the hardened chocolate bar into small squares and roll them around in the bowl. Add the quark, fromage frais, cornflour, egg, baking powder, vanilla extract and remaining powdered sweetener.

Line a baking sheet with aluminium foil and arrange the mixture in small piles, spacing them out evenly, and bake in the preheated oven for 20 minutes. Keep a careful eye on the biscuits until they are cooked.

CRUNCHY ALMOND BISCUITS
(BISCUITS CROQUANTS À L'AMANDE)

Preparation time: 30 minutes
Cooking time: 20 minutes
Makes approx. 30 biscuits

4 tablespoons oat bran
2 tablespoons wheat bran
1 tablespoon cornflour
15g (½oz) virtually fat-free quark
15g (½oz) fat-free fromage frais
2 eggs
2 teaspoons baking powder
1 teaspoon bitter almond flavouring
   (www.mydukandietshop.co.uk)
2 tablespoons powdered sweetener

Preheat the oven to 180°C/350°F/Gas 4.

In a bowl, mix together the oat bran, wheat bran, corn-flour, quark, fromage frais, eggs and baking powder. Then add the bitter almond flavouring and powdered sweetener. Spoon out approximately 30 biscuits on to a baking tray lined with foil or greaseproof paper, leaving enough space between them. Bake in the middle of the preheated oven for 20 minutes. Keep a careful eye on the biscuits as they cook. When they are done, take them out of the oven and leave them on the baking sheet to cool. Only remove them once they are cold.

CRUNCHY CAPPUCCINO COOKIES
(COOKIES CROQUANTS PARFUM CAPPUCCINO)

Preparation time: 40 minutes
Cooking time: 20 minutes
Makes 20–25 biscuits

4 tablespoons oat bran
2 tablespoons wheat bran
2 tablespoons cornflour
15g (½oz) virtually fat-free quark
15g (½oz) fat-free fromage frais
150g (5½oz) fat-free natural yoghurt
2 eggs
½ × 8g sachet baking powder
1 teaspoon instant coffee
4 tablespoons powdered sweetener
2 tablespoons skimmed milk powder

Preheat the oven to 160°C/325°F/Gas 3.

Combine all the ingredients thoroughly in a bowl. Line a baking tray with greaseproof paper. Spoon out 20–25 biscuits on to the tray, leaving enough space between them. Bake in the middle of the preheated oven for 20 minutes. Keep a careful eye on the biscuits as they cook and only remove them from the tray once they are cold.

RUM AND OAT BRAN CREAM
(CRÈME AU RHUM ET AU SON D'AVOINE)

Preparation time: 30 minutes
Cooking time: 5–10 minutes
6 servings

2 gelatine leaves
1 vanilla pod
500ml (18fl oz) skimmed milk
2 egg yolks
2 tablespoons powdered sweetener
4 tablespoons oat bran
1 teaspoon white or dark rum flavouring (www.
    mydukandietshop.co.uk)

Soak the gelatine leaves in some cold water for 5 minutes. Split the vanilla pod and scrape out the seeds into a pan with the milk. Bring to the boil then remove from the heat.

In a bowl, whisk together the egg yolks, sweetener, oat bran and rum flavouring. Pour the milk very carefully over the egg mixture, stirring continuously. Warm the mixture through without letting it boil – it should thicken slightly. Remove from the heat, add the gelatine and stir very thoroughly. Pour into glass dishes, leave to cool to room temperature then refrigerate for 4 hours before serving.

RHUBARB CRUMBLE
(CRUMBLE DE RHUBARBE)

Preparation time: 20 minutes
Cooking time: 40–45 minutes
1 serving

250g (9oz) rhubarb, cut into small chunks
Powdered sweetener, to taste
3 tablespoons oat bran
1 tablespoons wheat bran
1 egg white
1 tablespoon fat-free fromage frais

Preheat the oven to 200°C/400°F/Gas 6.

Gently cook the rhubarb, adding a little sweetener so that it tastes less bitter. In a bowl, combine the brans, egg white and fromage frais.

Reduce the oven temperature to 180°C/350°F/Gas 4 and line a baking sheet with greaseproof paper. Spread the crumble mixture over it and bake for 20 minutes. Once cooked, cut the mixture into small pieces and put in a blender. Bake the crumbs in the oven for a further 5 minutes.

In the meantime, pour the rhubarb into a ramekin dish then add the crumble topping when ready. Bake for another 10 minutes.

PISTACHIO SPONGE FINGERS
(FINANCIERS À LA PISTACHE)

Preparation time: 10 minutes
Cooking time: 5 minutes
Makes 4 sponge fingers

2 tablespoons oat bran
1 tablespoon wheat bran
2 egg whites
1 teaspoon pistachio flavouring (www.
    mydukandietshop.co.uk)
5 drops butter flavouring (www.mydukandietshop.
    co.uk)
1½ tablespoons powdered sweetener
1 teaspoon bitter almond flavouring (www.
    mydukandietshop.co.uk)
4 drops green food colouring
1 level teaspoon baking powder
1 tablespoon fat-free fromage frais
2 teaspoons cornflour

Preheat the oven to 180°C/350°F/Gas 4.

Blend the oat and wheat brans as finely as possible then put to one side. In a bowl, using an electric whisk, whizz together the egg whites, pistachio flavouring, butter flavouring, sweetener, bitter almond flavouring and food colouring until the eggs are nice and frothy. Add the baking powder, the fromage frais, cornflour and bran mix, and whisk for a further minute. Put the mixture into a finger biscuit mould, preferably a silicone one (about 1½ tablespoonfuls for each sponge finger). Turn the oven temperature down to 140°C/275°F/Gas 1 and bake on the middle shelf for 5 minutes. Keep a careful eye on the fingers until they are ready.

CHOCOLATE GALETTE
(GALETTE AU CHOCOLAT)

Preparation time: 5 minutes
Cooking time: 2–3 minutes
1 serving

1 sweet Dukan galette (see p.106)
1 egg yolk
1 teaspoon fat-reduced cocoa powder
Powdered sweetener, to taste

Make a sweet galette following the recipe on p.106. Combine the egg yolk and cocoa powder, adding a little sweetener until the mixture is to your taste. When it is, spread it all over the galette.

TIP As a tasty variation on this recipe, you can sprinkle cinnamon and aniseeds over the chocolate spread.

DOUBLE BRAN CAKE
(GÂTEAU AUX DEUX SONS)

Preparation time: 5 minutes
Cooking time: 40 minutes
4 servings

4 tablespoons wheat bran
8 tablespoons oat bran
2 egg whites
4 tablespoons fat-free fromage frais
2 teaspoons bitter almond flavouring (www.
    mydukandietshop.co.uk)
4 tablespoons powdered sweetener (for baking)
1 × 8g sachet baking powder
4 eggs

Preheat the oven to 180°C/350°F/Gas 4.

In a bowl, combine all the ingredients until the mixture is smooth and pour into a silicone cake tin, 20cm (8in) long, and bake for about 40 minutes.

VANILLA AND BLUEBERRY CAKE
(GÂTEAU LÉGER VANILLA ET MYRTILLES)

Preparation time: 25 minutes
Cooking time: 45 minutes
6 servings

4 eggs, separated, whites stiffly beaten
4 tablespoons powdered sweetener, to taste
1 teaspoon dark rum flavouring (www.
  · mydukandietshop.co.uk)
300g (10½oz) fat-free vanilla flavoured yoghurt
150g (5½oz) fat-free natural yoghurt
4 tablespoons oat bran
2 tablespoons wheat bran
2 tablespoons cornflour
3 large handfuls of blueberries, washed and dried

Preheat the oven to 150°C/300°F/Gas 2.

In a large bowl, whisk together the egg yolks with the sweetener and dark rum flavouring. Add both yoghurts and stir in thoroughly. Next fold in the two brans, the cornflour and the stiffly beaten egg whites, folding them in so that plenty of air gets into the mixture. Next add the blueberries.

Pour the mixture into a cake tin, preferably a silicone mould, and bake in the preheated oven for 45 minutes. The cake will rise but then sink slightly once removed from the oven.

CRUNCHY-FONDANT OAT BRAN MACAROONS (MACARONS CROUSTI-FONDANTS AU SON D'AVOINE)

Preparation time: 1 hour
Cooking time: 10 minutes
Makes 25 macaroons

2 tablespoons oat bran
1 teaspoon bitter almond flavouring (www.
 mydukandietshop.co.uk
2 tablespoons powdered sweetener
2 egg whites, stiffly beaten

Preheat the oven to 180°C/350°F/Gas 4 and line a baking tray with some foil.

Carefully fold the oat bran, bitter almond flavouring and powdered sweetener into the stiffly beaten egg whites, using a spatula to combine the ingredients without breaking up the egg whites. Take a piping bag or make one by snipping off the corner of a freezer bag. Pour in the mixture and shape about 25 small macaroons on the prepared baking tray. Reduce the oven temperature to 150°C/300°F/Gas 2 and bake for 10 minutes.. Keep a watchful eye on the macaroons if you have a glass-fronted oven but do not open the oven door while they are cooking. When they are done – the bottoms will have turned brown – switch the oven off and leave to cool for 30 minutes. Remove the macaroons from the tray once they are completely cold.

BUTTER MADELEINES
(MADELEINES AU BEURRE)

Preparation time: 5 minutes
Cooking time: 5 minutes
Makes 12 madeleines

2 tablespoons oat bran
1 tablespoon wheat bran
2 eggs
½ teaspoon lemon flavouring (www.
    mydukandietshop.co.uk)
20 drops butter flavouring (www.mydukandietshop.
    co.uk)
2 tablespoons powdered sweetener
2 tablespoons skimmed milk powder
2 teaspoons baking powder

Preheat the oven to 180°C/ 350°F/ Gas 4.

Whizz the oat bran and wheat bran in a blender and then keep to one side. Next blend the eggs, lemon flavouring, butter flavouring and powdered sweetener for 1 minute. Now add the skimmed milk powder, the bran mix and baking powder and blend for a further minute. If possible use a silicone mould and 1 table-spoon of the mixture for each madeleine. Turn the oven down to 140°C/275°F/Gas 1 and bake the madeleines on the middle shelf for 5 minutes. Do keep a careful eye on them as they cook very quickly!

TIP If you do not have a silicone mould, put your mould in the freezer while preparing the madeleine mixture.

LEMON MUFFINS
(MUFFINS AU CITRON)

Preparation time: 5 minutes
Cooking time: 15–20 minutes
2 servings

2 tablespoons oat bran
1 tablespoon wheat bran
4 tablespoons skimmed milk powder
1 egg
1 egg white
1 teaspoon lemon flavouring (www.mydukandietshop.
  co.uk)
1 teaspoon baking powder
1–2 tablespoons powdered sweetener

Preheat the oven to 180°C/350°F/Gas 4.

Blend the oat and wheat bran until as fine as possible. In a bowl, combine the blended bran with the remaining ingredients. Pour the mixture into two ramekin dishes and bake in the preheated oven for 15–20 minutes, keeping a careful eye on the muffins until they are ready.

ANTI-HUNGER PANCAKE
(PANCAKE COUPE-FAIM)

Preparation time: 5 minutes
Cooking time: 1 minute
1 serving

1 tablespoon wheat bran
2 tablespoons oat bran
4 tablespoons skimmed milk powder
1 egg
1 egg white
1 teaspoon vanilla flavouring (www.mydukandietshop.
   co.uk)
10 drops orange flower water
1–2 tablespoons powdered sweetener

In a bowl, combine all the ingredients. Using some
kitchen paper, lightly oil a non-stick frying pan and
cook the pancake for 30 seconds on each side, using a
spatula to flip it over.

MINT AND TEA FLAVOURED PUFF BISCUITS (PETITS COUSSINS AU THÉ ET À LA MENTHE)

Preparation time: 10 minutes
Cooking time: 20 minutes
1 serving

2 tablespoons oat bran
2 teaspoons finely chopped dried mint
½ teaspoon Matcha green tea powder
4 tablespoons skimmed milk powder
1 teaspoon baking powder
1 teaspoon powdered sweetener
1 egg, beaten
1 egg white

Preheat the oven to 180°C/350°F/Gas 4.

Whizz the oat bran in a blender then stir in the finely chopped mint, tea powder, powdered milk, baking powder and sweetener. Add the beaten egg and the egg white, and mix. Divide the mixture between two ramekins and bake in the preheated oven for 20 minutes.

CHOCOLATE AND PISTACHIO CAKES (PETITS GÂTEAUX PISTACHE-CHOCOLAT)

Preparation time: 10 minutes
Cooking time: 20 minutes
2 servings

3 tablespoons oat bran
2 tablespoons skimmed milk powder
2 eggs, separated
1 tablespoon cornflour
1 teaspoon pistachio flavouring (www.
   mydukandietshop.co.uk)
1 teaspoon baking powder
4 drops green food colouring
5 tablespoons powdered sweetener
1 teaspoon fat-reduced cocoa powder
½ teaspoon rum

Preheat the oven to 180°C/350°F/Gas 4. Using a drop of oil on some kitchen paper lightly oil two non-stick cake moulds.

In a bowl, combine the oat bran, milk powder, egg whites, cornflour, pistachio flavouring, baking powder, food colouring and 3 tablespoons of the powdered sweetener, then put to one side. In another bowl, mix together the egg yolks, cocoa powder, the remaining powdered sweetener and the rum.

Half-fill the prepared moulds with the pistachio

mixture, then carefully add the cocoa mixture on top, finishing off with the rest of the pistachio mixture (do not fill the moulds right to the top as the cakes will expand). Bake in the preheated oven for 20 minutes, keeping a careful eye on them at the end.

OAT BRAN PORRIDGE

Preparation time: 2 minutes
Cooking time: 6–7 minutes
1 serving

200ml (7fl oz) skimmed milk
1 teaspoon vanilla flavouring
3 tablespoons oat bran
Powdered sweetener, to taste

In a pan, heat the skimmed milk with the vanilla flavouring. Add the oat bran and stir until it becomes nice and thick. Remove from the heat and add the sweetener. Eat either hot or cold.

RHUBARB SPONGE
(PUDDING À LA RHUBARBE)

Preparation time: 30 minutes
Cooking time: 40 minutes
4 servings

For the sponge
2 tablespoons oat bran
1 tablespoon wheat bran
2 generous teaspoons baking powder
10 drops vanilla flavouring (www.mydukandietshop.
    co.uk)
8 drops butter flavouring (www.mydukandietshop.co.uk)
5 drops white rum flavouring (www.mydukandietshop.
    co.uk)
Cinnamon
6 tablespoons skimmed milk powder
4 tablespoons fat-free fromage frais
2 tablespoons powdered sweetener

For the cream
2 large or 3 medium egg yolks
3 tablespoons powdered sweetener
300ml (10fl oz) milk

For the topping
115g (4oz) rhubarb compote or jam
50g (1¾oz) rhubarb chunks (cooked with sweetener)

Prepare the sponge as you would a sweet white bread loaf, combining the oat and wheat brans, baking powder, flavourings, some cinnamon, the skimmed milk powder, fromage frais and sweetener. Divide the mixture between two containers of the same size and bake each one in turn for 3–4 minutes in the microwave (or both at once for 5 minutes). Leave to cool a little.

Preheat the oven to 180°C/ 350°F/ Gas 4.

Prepare the cream: in a bowl, whisk together the egg yolks and the sweetener. Heat the milk in a pan and then gently pour it over the eggs. Stir thoroughly and return the mixture to the pan. Keep stirring until it thickens and resembles custard.

Take each 'loaf' and split it in two lengthways. Spread each half with the rhubarb compote or jam then cut them up to make strips roughly a finger's width.

Cover the bottom of a cake tin with the strips, the rhubarb facing upwards, and add a few chunks of the cooked fruit. Pour half the cream over. Wait 5–10 minutes for the sponge to absorb some of the cream then cover it with the rest of the strips – this time the rhubarb should face downwards. Finish off with the remaining cream and sprinkle with a little cinnamon. Bake in the preheated oven in a bain-marie for 40 minutes. Leave to cool to room temperature before serving.

CINNAMON TART
(TARTE À LA CANNELLE)

Preparation time: 25 minutes
Cooking time: 40 minutes
4 servings

Powdered sweetener, to taste
3 eggs, beaten
1 tablespoon ground cinnamon
250g (9oz) virtually fat-free quark and fat-free fromage frais
1 vanilla pod
1 quantity sweet Dukan galette dough (see p.106)

Preheat the oven to 220°C/425°F/Gas 7 and line a flan dish with baking paper.

First prepare the filling by beating the sweetener into the eggs until the mixture takes on a creamy consistency. Next fold in the cinnamon, quark and fromage frais. Split open the vanilla pod, scrape out the seeds and add them to the mixture.

Make the sweet galette dough following the recipe on p.106 and use this as your pastry base. Press the dough into the prepared dish and bake in the preheated oven for 10 minutes. Pour in the filling and bake for a further 30 minutes.

Acknowledgements

To Sylvia.

One day when I was 13 my mother took me to one side and, placing her hand on my head, she said these few very simple words to me:

'Pierre, my son, listen to me carefully. You are young, you enjoy good health, you are bright and you were born into a well-off family, and you are part of a big family that loves you. You go to school and you seem to be doing well. You are a handsome chap. This is an awful lot for just one person, can you see that? So, when you are grown up, try to give a little of this back to those people who have not had all this.'

I first want to thank the woman who brought me into this world, who gave me life and showed me the pleasure of giving others pleasure.

Many people have made it possible for me to write this book but I would like to thank Carol in particular, whose help and expertise are only surpassed by her modesty.

My thanks also go to Anna for her support and understanding.

I also want to thank my wife and children for allowing me to spend all these hours writing when I should have been enjoying their company.

And thanks to life for being alive!

INDEX

Index

Index

Index

vanilla
  anti-hunger pancake 169
  chocolate chip biscuits 154–5
  flavouring in galettes 104, 110
  oat bran porridge 173
  rhubarb sponge 174–5
  rum and oat bran cream 158
  vanilla and blueberry cake 164
vegetables, tinned 91–2
vitamin absorption 28–9

weight gain 8–9
  and insulin 24, 81–2
  suffering caused by 56
weight loss
  finding pleasure in 48–51,
    55–6, 57

  and lifestyle 42
  and oat bran 89
  rapid 41
  Stabilization weight 32–3
wheat bran 101
  and constipation 95
  as insoluble fibre 14, 15
women
  and cancer 88
  and constipation 94, 95

yoghurt
  vanilla and blueberry cake 164

Discover the complete Dukan Diet collection

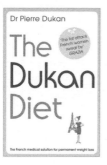

The Dukan Diet

The original and bestselling diet

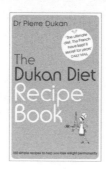

The Dukan Diet Recipe Book

350 essential Dukan recipes

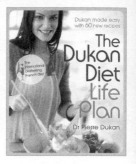

The Dukan Diet Life Plan

Dukan made easy, including 60 recipes, in full colour

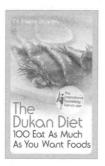

The Dukan Diet 100 Eat As Much As You Want Foods

The ultimate guide to the 100 Dukan-friendly foods

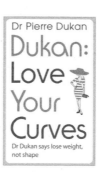

Love Your Curves

Dr Dukan's personal message that we should lose weight, not shape

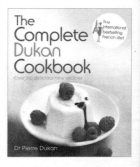

The Complete Dukan Cookbook

350 Dukan recipes, with full colour photographs